INSIDE FORENSIC SCIENCE

The Forensic Aspects of Poisons

INSIDE FORENSIC SCIENCE

Forensic Anthropology

Forensic DNA Analysis

Forensic Medicine

Forensic Pharmacology

Legal Aspects of Forensics

The Forensic Aspects of Poisons

INSIDE FORENSIC SCIENCE

The Forensic Aspects of Poisons

Richard A. Stripp, Ph.D.

SERIES EDITOR | Lawrence Kobilinsky, Ph.D.

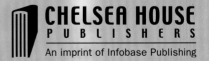
CHELSEA HOUSE
PUBLISHERS
An imprint of Infobase Publishing

Chelsea House
An imprint of Infobase Publishing
132 West 31st Street
New York NY 10001

ISBN-10: 0-7910-9197-X
ISBN-13: 978-0-7910-9197-5

Library of Congress Cataloging-in-Publication Data
Stripp, Richard A.
    The Forensic aspects of poisons / Richard A. Stripp.
        p. cm. — (Inside forensic science)
    Includes bibliographical references (p.) and index.
    ISBN 0-7910-9197-X (hardcover)
    1. Forensic toxicology. I. Title. II. Series.
RA1228.S77 2006
614ʹ.13—dc22

                                                    2006022825

Chelsea House books are available at special discounts when purchased in bulk quantities for businesses, associations, institutions, or sales promotions. Please call our Special Sales Department in New York at (212) 967-8800 or (800) 322-8755.

You can find Chelsea House on the World Wide Web at http://www.chelseahouse.com

Cover design by Ben Peterson
Text design by Annie O'Donnell
Printed in the United States of America

Bang FOF 10 9 8 7 6 5 4 3 2

This book is printed on acid-free paper.

All links and Web addresses were checked and verified to be correct at the time of publication. Because of the dynamic nature of the Web, some addresses and links may have changed since publication and may no longer be valid.

Table of Contents

Introduction to the Science of Poisons

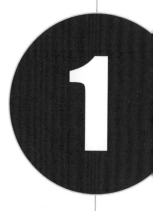

All substances are poisons; there is none which is not a poison.
The right dose differentiates a poison from a remedy.
—Paracelsus (1493–1541)

The history of *forensic toxicology* goes back approximately 200 years. Toxicology is defined as the study of poisons, but it also covers the detection and measurement of chemicals, such as alcohol, drugs, poisonous gases, and industrial chemicals, in biological specimens, including human tissues and remains. Sometimes a toxicological analysis may involve a blood, urine, or hair sample from a living person. The widely used method of determining blood alcohol by testing a person's breath is an example of an application in clinical forensic toxicology (Figure 1.1). In postmortem toxicology (analysis of a deceased person), an **autopsy** is required in which tissue samples and body fluids are tested for poisons or drugs.

WHAT IS A POISON?

A **poison** is any agent capable of producing harm in a living organism. All chemicals have the potential to be poisons if

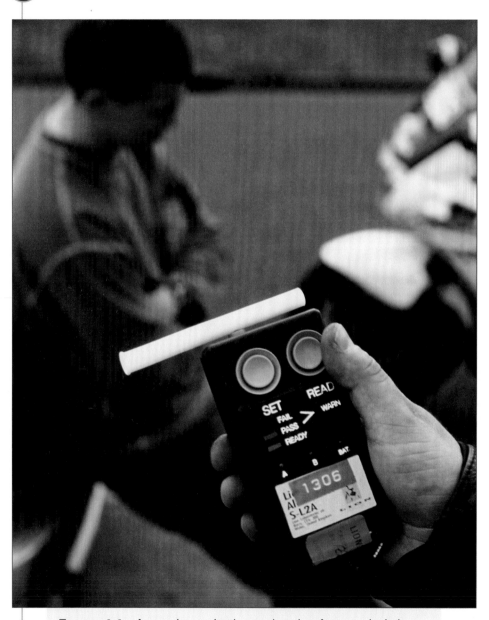

FIGURE 1.1 A motorist awaits the results taken from an alcohol breath test. A breathalyzer indicates the blood alcohol content (BAC) in one's breath, thus determining whether a person has been driving under the influence of alcohol. In most states, it is illegal to drive with a BAC of .08% or higher.

present in sufficient amount. However, the toxicity of chemicals varies: 0.00001 milligrams (mg) of botulinum toxin per kilogram (kg) of body weight may be acutely lethal in an animal, while ethyl alcohol requires 10,000 mg/kg to produce death. Therefore, botulinum toxin (the cause of botulism) is 10 billion times more **toxic** than alcohol. So, although all things may be poisonous, not all poisons have the same potential to cause harm. However, from a forensic perspective, alcohol is the most abused drug in the world and contributes to thousands of deaths; overall, its effects are felt far more than botulinum toxin. There are many factors to consider when assessing the overall impact of a drug or chemical on society.

We can classify toxic agents by looking at their target organs, use, source, and effects. They may be classified according to their physical state, chemical reactivity, structure, or poisoning potential. Toxins or venoms are poisons produced by living organisms, such as plants, bacteria, fungi, and venomous animals. Man-made poisonous agents are called toxicants and include environmental pollutants, industrial and household chemicals, and many drugs.

POISONING IN HISTORY

Knowledge of toxic venoms from animals and plants is something that predates any historical record. Early man quickly learned which snakes to avoid and the particular plants he should not consume due to their dangerous nature. Even early written history is rich in descriptions of poisons and practices related to toxicology. The Ebers papyrus (circa 1500 B.C.) contains writings about toxins such as opium, metals, and hemlock. The Bible also has references to poison arrows (The book of Job, circa 1400 B.C.). Ancient Greek teachings of Hippocrates (460–377 B.C.) and others contain numerous references to poisons as well. During the time of the Roman Empire, poisoning someone as a way to commit murder gained legendary popularity, giving rise to such thankless careers as food tasters.

For centuries, poisoning has been a popular way to do away with a known rival. History has shown poisoning to be the method of choice for women who want to commit murder, perhaps due to the perceived nonviolent nature of the act. Little or no blood is shed, poisoning often mimics a natural disease, and the victims often do not know they are being poisoned. However, the demographics have changed somewhat, and males are now just as likely to murder by poison. Almost any natural substance in the right dose can be toxic and many cause symptoms that are nonspecific, appearing to be common diseases, leading to the belief that the victim died of natural causes.

From the poisoners of ancient Rome, carrying out their deadly practice in planned secret, to the possibility of the use of chemical weapons by terrorists, society must always confront the role of toxic substances in criminal activities. Film and television have popularized the image of a clever, murderous individual deliberately poisoning another in a homicidal and evil confrontation (Figure 1.2). Some may envision the legend of Cleopatra dying as a result of a bite from a poisonous snake (although most historians believe Cleopatra's death by poison was a suicide and not a homicide). Ancient humanity learned quite quickly that exposure to certain substances resulted in very negative outcomes. Perhaps the observation of someone becoming very ill and possibly dying after eating a certain plant or mineral was the event from which the early poisoners learned to practice their deadly trade.

Poisoning for criminal purposes receives little attention except when it is sensationalized by media tabloids or involves a celebrity. Although poisonings account for fewer than 10% of homicides,

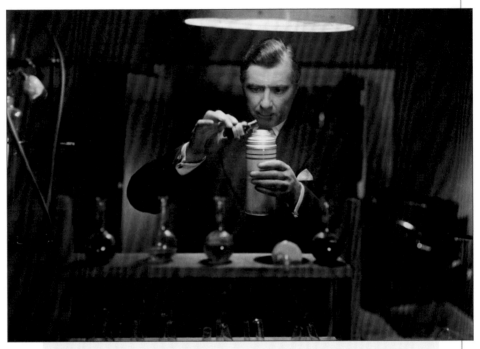

FIGURE 1.2 Actor Robert Newton prepares a poisonous drink in the 1949 film *Obsession*. Newton plays a deranged doctor who intends to murder his wife's lover.

many cases of criminal poisoning may go undetected due to problems associated with identifying this type of crime. Sometimes when suspicious evidence surfaces later on, the case involves the unearthing of the victim's remains from the burial site. There are problems, however, with detecting poisons in a body that has been **embalmed** and buried. For many reasons, poisoning cases can be missed in the initial investigation process—it has even been joked that toxicologists bury their mistakes.

While it has been practiced for centuries, the use of poison is a unique method of crime. Poisonings often involve passionate and vengeful types of murder and require a methodical, cunning, and devious criminal. He or she usually plans the act in

advance, and frequently the crime requires repetitive administration of the poison. Because the crime is one of premeditation,
there are no examples of poisoning in self-defense. Given such
facts, the crime of **homicidal poisoning** would seem to be a
popular area of study, but there are few studies related to the history of poisoning and the nature of poisoners and their victims.
Yet, the potential for toxic substances to become weapons of
mass destruction has increased dramatically in recent years. The
patterns of poisoning are critical to assisting law enforcement
professionals in their preparedness in the unthinkable event of a
mass poisoning. Studies are needed to develop an understanding
of the characteristics of such a crime.

CHARACTERISTICS OF POISONING CASES

The investigation of poisoning cases relies on victim and
poisoner characteristics, as well as cooperation between the
medical and law enforcement communities. Studies show that
victims of homicidal poisonings are divided almost equally
between males and females and the victims' ages range from
less than one week old to 75 years or older. The greatest number
of victims falls in the age range from 25 to 44 years old. When
victims are female, the offenders are predominantly male. In
contrast, if victims are male, the offenders are divided almost
equally between males and females. The poisoner is predominantly white and the offender is usually the same race as the
victim. Additional findings show that white victims are predominantly the targets of male poisoners, blacks are almost
equally the victims of male and female offenders, and people
of other racial backgrounds are equally likely to be victims of
female or unknown offenders.

Recently, it has been shown that 48.6% of the poisoners in the
1990s were male, compared with 33.2% female offenders, which

would seem to challenge the perception that mostly women use poisons. Of course, these cases represented only those murders that became known to law enforcement. It may be that women are more likely to be poisoners, but are better at getting away with the crime. The poisoners' ages ranged from 10 years to 75 years or older. The age range of 20 to 34 years accounted for 32% of the criminals. Since the percent of poisoners with unknown characteristics is said to be 20 to 30 times higher than those with unknown characteristics among all murderers, some of these demographic findings must remain tentative. This problem is most likely due to a lack of witnesses, which commonly occurs with poisoning; therefore, little information is available regarding many of these crimes.

Every death may be considered a homicide until proven otherwise, and every death with no visible signs of injury or obvious cause for death may be considered a possible poisoning. The investigation of a homicidal poisoning involves examining the potential clues and developing a list of possible suspects. The classic scenario of identifying the victim, finding the poison and determining how it was administered, examining the crime scene, and establishing motive are all necessary pieces to the puzzle.

THE IMPORTANCE OF FORENSIC TOXICOLOGY

Forensic toxicology is important not just for when criminal activity is suspected but also for determining the role of drugs and chemicals in accidental deaths and suicides. Forensic toxicologists are often called upon to figure out what part drugs may play in the commission of a crime, in accidents or violent deaths (such as car accidents), and in substance abuse while on the job or at school. A toxicologist may be asked to test for substances ranging from toxic metals, cyanide, carbon monoxide, alcohol, and abused drugs to prescribed or over-the-counter drugs. According to the American Chemical Society, there are about 21 million registered compounds—quite a daunting task for the forensic toxicologist! This book will allow you to experience how the toxicologist deals with this seemingly overwhelming mission.

Modern Forensic Toxicology

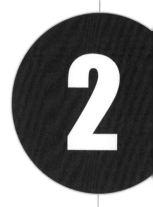

There are no such things as applied sciences, only applications of science.

—Louis Pasteur (1822–1895)

The founding father of forensic toxicology was a physician named Orfila, who developed the art of chemical analysis and applied it to the investigation of criminal poisoning. It was the testimony by Professor Orfila in the 1840 homicide-by-arsenic trial of Madame Lafarge that is often credited with bringing the science of forensic toxicology into the criminal courts, and thus planting the seeds of modern toxicology.

Early in the development of the field, forensic toxicologists were considered to be coroners' chemists, who were limited to the application of routine laboratory benchwork. During the last few decades, this view has changed. The forensic toxicologist must determine what and how much poisonous substance is present in human tissue samples and interpret these results through an understanding of the episode of intoxication. Academic programs in forensic toxicology were once few but are now found in several universities in the United States.

Forensic toxicologists are very much like scientific detectives (Figure 2.1). Since poisons continue to be named as causes of death and disease, forensic toxicologists must continue to carry out their job as seekers of the truth. As technology advances, toxicologists continue to adopt highly sensitive, modern analytical methods to investigate the role of chemicals in causing illness and death.

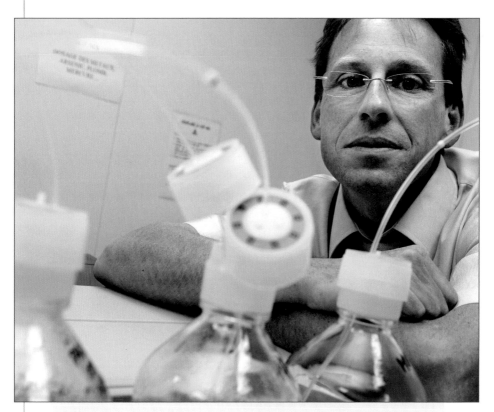

FIGURE 2.1 Toxicologist and forensic specialist Pascal Kintz played detective in 2001 when he proved that French emperor Napoleon Bonaparte died of arsenic poisoning rather than stomach cancer, which is listed as the cause of death on his death certificate. Kintz conducted a chemical analysis on a lock of hair preserved after Napoleon's death, which revealed a higher than normal concentration of arsenic.

TYPES OF INVESTIGATIONS

Forensics is the application of many different fields of science to the legal system. This may involve criminal activity or civil actions. Forensic toxicology is a field of forensics that applies the principles of toxicology to legal purposes. It includes three major categories: postmortem toxicology, human performance toxicology, and forensic drug testing. Early forensic toxicology dealt with only postmortem investigations, but today forensic toxicologists are involved in a variety of cases. All work or opinions of the toxicologist must withstand the scrutiny of a court of law. Reports and findings may be introduced as evidence and the toxicologist is often asked to testify. A forensic toxicologist must consider all aspects of an investigation, such as any possible symptoms, evidence found at a crime scene, or any relevant information related to the history of a case. Armed with this information and samples for analysis, the forensic toxicologist determines what toxic substances may be related to the case and at what concentrations they are present. He or she must then interpret the probable role that a drug or poison played in the case.

TOXIC AGENTS

Many toxic substances do not produce any overt lesions, so in the absence of other suspect causes of death or injury, a toxic reaction may be suspected. Since all things are potentially toxic, these agents can exist in several forms: gases, liquids, or solids that can be of animal (e.g., biological toxins), mineral (e.g., metals), or vegetable origins. They can be therapeutic or abused drugs, venoms, household and industrial chemicals, environmental pollutants, or naturally occurring substances, to name but a few. The routes of exposure include inhalation, ingestion, injection, and absorption through the skin.

Metabolite

They can enter the body in a single, large dose or in smaller doses over time. The concentrations found in the body can range from trace (almost not detectable) amounts to larger quantities.

Some toxins may be detected intact, but the body quickly transforms others into new compounds called **metabolites.** This means that a toxicologist must test for metabolites of a toxin, perhaps in addition to the toxin itself. For example, heroin is almost immediately metabolized into morphine and other metabolites, which can be readily detected, while the heroin content is rapidly reduced and more difficult to detect.

Poisonous Spiders

A 21-year-old otherwise healthy man presented with severe abdominal and groin pain. Upon arrival at the emergency room, he was agitated and complaining of severe pain. Upon further questioning, he said that he had been bitten on the toe by a black spider 2 hours before the pain began. He was treated and his symptoms lasted for 24 hours. He was discharged 36 hours after the bite.

At Halloween, spiders hang from every window and lurk behind every door. Which ones might make you fret? Black widow and brown recluse spiders are the two spider species in the United States that most commonly send their victims to the emergency room. Black widow spiders (*Latrodectus mactans*) are found in all states except Alaska. They inhabit warm, dark, and dry places. The underbelly of the spider frequently has a distinctive red hourglass marking. Although folklore suggests that only the female black widow has venom, the male spider also has venom but its

CAUSES OF DEATH

Certainly, the role the forensic toxicologist plays is quite daunting. The number of deaths and injuries related to drugs, alcohol, and poisons is highly significant.

- About 3 in every 10 Americans will be involved in an alcohol-related traffic accident at some time in their lives. Motor vehicle crashes are the leading cause of death for people 33 years old or younger.

- There were an estimated 5,800 pedestrian deaths and 90,000 injuries in the year 2000. Bicycling resulted in

small teeth prevent it from penetrating human skin. The principal agent in the venom is a neurotoxin. Following a bite the victim may feel an initial pricking sensation followed in one to two hours by lymph node tenderness. The site may be surrounded by a white area with a thin swollen ring around the bite. Muscle cramping in the affected extremity may be severe. Depending on the location of the bite, cramping may also affect muscles in the abdomen, chest, or back. Other symptoms include nausea, vomiting, sweating, hypertension, and elevated heart rate. Pain may start as early as 20 minutes following a bite but often does not start for 2 to 3 hours and frequently comes and goes. Significant symptoms often last for 36 to 72 hours, but the time course and severity are quite variable. The pain may be excruciating and can be mistaken for a heart attack, especially when the spider bite is not reported to the attending physician.

about 800 deaths due to collisions with motor vehicles in which alcohol and drugs played a significant role.

- The four leading fatal events are poisonings, falls, fires and burns, and suffocation by an ingested object.

- The leading cause of death in the home, poisoning, took the lives of 11,500 people in 2001. This number includes deaths from drugs, medicines, other solid and liquid substances, and gases and vapors. The 25 to 44 age group had the highest death rate.

- Falls took the lives of 9,000 people, 4 out of 5 of them over the age of 65 in the year 2000.

- Smoke inhalation (carbon monoxide and cyanide poisoning) accounts for the preponderance of deaths in home fires, and alcohol is detected in a large majority of victims in such cases.

- Recreational boating resulted in 701 deaths in 2000. Alcohol was reported to be involved in 31% of these deaths.

- Each year, use of NSAIDs (nonsteroidal anti-inflammatory drugs) accounts for an estimated 7,600 deaths and 76,000 hospitalizations in the United States. NSAIDs include aspirin, ibuprofen, and naproxen.

- Illicit drug use is associated with suicide, homicide, car accidents, HIV infection, pneumonia, violence, mental illness, and hepatitis. It is estimated that more than 3 million individuals in the United States have serious drug problems.

Source: Mokdad, A.H., J.S. Marks, D.F. Stroup, and J.L. Gerberding. "Actual Causes of Death in the United States." Journal of the American Medical Association 291, no. 10 (March 10, 2004): 1238-1245.

Due to the lack of proper reporting, the exact number of poisonings in the United States is not known. The leading cause of fatal injury across all age groups and for both sexes is motor vehicle crashes and as many as 50% of these are alcohol- and drug-related. The number one cause of nonfatal injuries is falls and, again, alcohol is a significant contributor. Violence-related deaths also rank high among the leading causes of death, and

Table 2.1 Causes of Death in the United States in 2000 Related to Poison, Drugs, or Alcohol

CAUSE OF DEATH	NUMBER (IN THOUSANDS)	PERCENT OF TOTAL DEATHS
Tobacco	435	18.1
Alcohol	85	3.5
Microbial agents	75	3.1
Toxic agents	55	2.3
Motor vehicle crash	26	1.2
Adverse reactions to prescription drugs	32	1.3
Suicide	30.6	1.3
Firearms incidents	29	1.2
Homicide	20	0.8
Sexual behaviors	20	0.8
Illicit drug use	17	0.7
Nonsteroidal anti-inflammatory drugs	7.6	0.3

Source: Substance Abuse and Mental Health Services Administration (SAMHSA). *National Survey on Drug Use and Health.*

drugs are known to contribute greatly to violent deaths. Females are much more likely than males to attempt suicide, with higher nonfatal self-harm injury rates; however, males are more likely to commit suicide. For females, suicide by poisoning is among the 10 leading causes of death.

About 2 million poisoning cases are officially documented each year. In the United States, fatalities from poisoning usually number in the tens of thousands each year. Of all poisonings reported, young children (under age 6) account for the largest percentage. However, adults account for the majority of fatal poisonings, with the greatest number of these being intentional (suicide) or accidental drug overdoses.

THE TOXICOLOGICAL INVESTIGATION

In a perfect world, we could categorize all substances as either toxic or nontoxic. However, as Paracelsus said, "All substances are poisons; there is none which is not a poison. The right dose differentiates a poison from a remedy." So, it is not really proper to say a substance is never toxic. However, we can still figure out the level of risk of exposure to a chemical based upon how toxic it is compared to other chemicals. People differ widely in their responses to many substances. Nonetheless, the forensic toxicologist is charged with detecting and keeping track of a large number of chemical agents in biological samples. The significance of the results must often be explained to a jury. The pharmacology, toxicology, local patterns of drug abuse, and postmortem changes can all affect the results. In any case, a good toxicologist must be prepared to answer the following questions:

1. What drug was taken, when, and how?
2. Was the drug or drugs sufficient to kill or to affect behavior?

3. Was a substance taken for therapeutic purposes, was it abused recreationally, was it used for suicidal purposes, or was it administered homicidally?
4. Was the person intoxicated at the time of the incident?
5. What are the effects on behavior or performance?
6. How would a person show intoxication with this substance?
7. Is there an alternative explanation for the findings?
8. What additional tests might shed light on these questions?

THE MODERN FORENSIC TOXICOLOGY LABORATORY

For an investigation, a forensic toxicologist receives samples of body fluids, tissues, and organs that are removed at autopsy. There will also be access to the case history, which may contain helpful information regarding possible symptoms of poisoning as well as other relevant pre- and postmortem information. In order to accurately interpret these findings, the toxicologist needs a thorough knowledge of how drugs and chemicals enter the body, what happens to them once they enter (i.e., how the body chemically transforms them), and how they are excreted.

The drugs must be separated and isolated from the tissues and potentially interfering substances must be removed. Most drugs are acidic or basic and they are separated from biological samples by acidic or basic **extraction.** Acidic drugs are extracted with an organic solvent at a pH solution of less than 7; basic drugs are extracted with a solution that has a pH greater than 7. Neutral drugs can be extracted at any pH. For example, cocaine is a basic drug that would be soluble in organic solvent at a basic pH, while **barbiturates** would be soluble at an acidic pH due to their acidic groups. Further details on proper collection, storage, and preparation of biological samples are discussed elsewhere in this book.

Following various sample preparation and separation techniques, forensic toxicological analysis consists of two major steps: **preliminary screening tests** and **confirmational analysis.** Confirmation is the use of methods that give structurally specific information about a compound in order to eliminate the potential for false positive results. Screening tests allow the toxicologist to rapidly test for a variety of drugs and toxins. Screening

	Table 2.2 Common Types of Poisoning	
RANK	**MOST FREQUENT REPORTED POISONING**	**MOST FREQUENT DEATH BY POISONING**
1	Household cleaning supplies	Antidepressant medications
2	Analgesics (aspirin, acetaminophen)	Analgesics (aspirin, acetaminophen)
3	Cosmetics	Drugs of abuse
4	Cough and cold remedies	Cardiovascular drugs
5	Toxic plants, animal and insect venoms	Alcohol
6	Pesticides	Gases and fumes (carbon monoxide)
7	Topical creams and lotions	Asthma therapies
8	Hydrocarbons (gasoline, kerosene)	Industrial chemicals
9	Antimicrobacterial soaps	Pesticides
10	Sedatives, hypnotics, antipsychotics	Household cleaning supplies
11	Food poisoning	Anticonvulsant medications
12	Alcohol	Food, plants, and insects

tests give preliminary results, and then a positive result must be verified with a confirmatory test.

TESTING FOR POISONS

Screening methods provide information regarding the presence of drugs or poisons. This may be relatively specific to a particular drug or poison or to a particular class of drugs. No single technique can detect everything, but a screening protocol should detect or eliminate as many substances as possible. Screening tests include immunoassays, chromatography, and color tests. Certain drugs and chemicals are more commonly encountered by the toxicologist (alcohol, cocaine, opiates, amphetamines, and **sedatives**), therefore specific screening tests will look for these substances. If a more exotic agent is suspected in a case, then additional tests may be requested. Often the nature of the poison is unidentified and termed a **general unknown**. In cases of this type, a full toxicology screen of all available specimens by several different techniques is required.

When a presumptive positive result is obtained for a substance, it must then be confirmed and quantified. Confirmation means obtaining analytic data from which it may be concluded with reasonable scientific certainty that a particular substance is present. This is necessary since presumptive positive findings may often be false positives due to interference in the test sample from contamination, improper handling, or the presence of other drugs. Confirmation tests look for structurally specific information about a compound in order to eliminate the potential for false positive results.

The most common technique used for confirmational analysis is gas chromatography/mass spectrometry (GC/MS). GC/MS combines gas-liquid chromatography for separation of the components and mass spectrometry to identify different substances

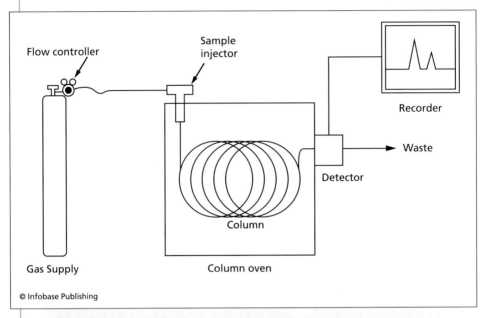

Flow controller

Sample injector

Recorder

Waste

Detector

Column

Gas Supply

Column oven

© Infobase Publishing

FIGURE 2.2 Schematic diagram of a gas chromatograph showing the major components.

within the test sample. In addition to drug detection, it is used for a variety of forensic applications, including seized drug analysis, arson and explosives investigations, and airport security to screen baggage for illicit substances. GC/MS is considered the best method for forensic substance identification and confirmational analysis.

In the GC/MS, the gas chromatograph separates the chemical components based on differences in their chemical properties (Figure 2.2). The result is that the molecules pass through the GC column at different rates, thus separating them based upon their individual retention times on the column. As the substances leave the gas chromatograph, they enter the mass spectrometer to be identified. The most common mass spectrometer uses a high-energy electron beam to break up the molecules and ionizes the sample material into fragments. Each molecule has an

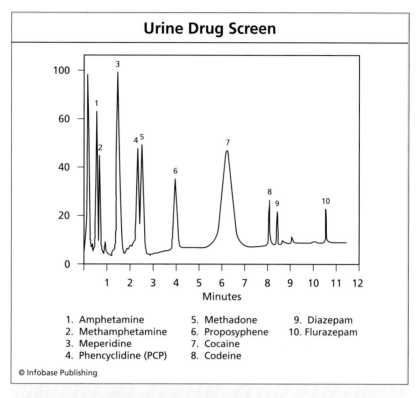

Urine Drug Screen

1. Amphetamine
2. Methamphetamine
3. Meperidine
4. Phencyclidine (PCP)
5. Methadone
6. Proposyphene
7. Cocaine
8. Codeine
9. Diazepam
10. Flurazepam

© Infobase Publishing

FIGURE 2.3 Typical chromatogram showing the separation of different drugs that may be detected in urine.

identifiable spectrum that can be compared by a computer to a library of thousands of spectra for a match (Figure 2.3). By using GC/MS, a very accurate identification is possible. The likelihood that two different samples could have the same retention time and the same spectra is near impossible. When a specific mass spectrum appears at a retention time for a particular compound, it is considered to be proof, with a very high degree of scientific certainty, that the particular molecule in the sample has been positively identified. Another widely used technique is liquid chromatography/mass spectrometry (LC/MS), in which the separation phase uses a liquid rather than a gas. Here the LC portion of the technique is used for preliminary separation of the components.

Qualitative analysis itself can only tell us what drug or poison was present. Information as to the possible role it played in a death or accident, or the person's level of intoxication, requires **quantitative analysis**. The samples used for this purpose are typically from blood, or the liver or other organs. Stomach contents may also be analyzed for total amount of drug present. Typically, quantities are determined by chromatography, either GC/MS or LC/MS.

TOXICOLOGY IN THE COURTROOM

The results of a toxicological investigation may be included in court testimony. Either the forensic pathologist or a qualified toxicologist may be asked to give an opinion as to whether a drug or toxin contributed to a death or accident or played a role

Table 2.3 Toxicological Screening and Confirmation Tests
SCREENING TESTS
Chemical spot tests: various color tests
Immunoassays: radioimmunoassay (RIA), fluorescent polarization immunoassay (FPIA), enzyme-multiplied immunoassay (EMIT), kinetic interaction of microparticles in solution immunoassay (KIMS), enzyme-linked immunosorbent assay (ELISA)
Chromatography: thin-layer, gas, high-performance liquid
Other: physical tests, crystal tests
CONFIRMATION TESTS
Gas chromatography/Mass spectrometry (GC/MS)
Liquid chromatography/Mass spectrometry (LC/MS)

in a violent crime. Often, the defense will call its own experts to dispute the opinions given by the plaintiff or prosecutor's medical experts. Cases involving drugs and toxins often become a battle of the experts and such proceedings can become quite intense, with the jury left to decide which expert opinion seems most likely to be true.

The following is a sampling of the types of questions that the forensic toxicologist might be asked by medical, legal, or law enforcement professionals:

- Was the driver intoxicated at the time of a car crash?

- Was a defendant under the influence of PCP (angel dust) when he shot and killed two acquaintances?

- Was cocaine-induced psychosis a likely explanation for a person's bizarre and violent behavior?

- Was alcohol involved when a person fell down a flight of stairs?

- (In the case of a death in a fire) Was the victim burned? Is the death consistent with smoke inhalation? Was the victim dead before the fire started?

- Were drugs used to incapacitate a girl during an alleged date rape?

- Was a drug used to commit suicide?

- Was a person murdered with a poison?

The forensic toxicologist must be able to provide accurate and concise answers to these questions using language that is easily understood by juries, judges, and lawyers. Furthermore, the opinions expressed by the toxicologist must always be impartial and based only on the scientific facts involved.

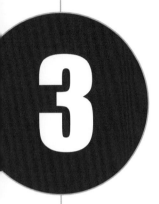

Types of Poisons

Never cry over spilt milk, because it may have been poisoned.
—W.C. Fields (1880–1946)

There are several definitions of what makes a poison a poison.
We already know that a poison is something that causes illness
and death. As stated earlier, any substance can be a poison if
taken in the right amount. This concept is at the very core of
toxicology: The dose is the key to determining the outcome of
exposure to a chemical.

Certainly, there are quantitative differences between substances in toxic potential. Cyanide is more toxic than aspirin,
but large quantities of aspirin can also be fatal. Some chemicals are more potent when it comes to toxicity and potential as
poisons, so we can make judgments about their relative safety
or hazardous nature. In addition, people differ widely in their
susceptibility to many drugs and poisons, depending on time of
usage, genetic predisposition, individual metabolism, preexisting medical conditions, and so on. What is fatal to one person
may be much less dangerous to another.

What makes a poison an efficient and deadly instrument of
murder? A poison used as a weapon needs to be toxic enough that

small quantities are effective; it should be easily disguised (in water or food); if it is to be administered orally, the taste or odor should be easily masked; it should cause symptoms that are delayed and nonspecific or appear to be due to natural illness; it must be readily obtainable and relatively easy to work with. This chapter looks at selected examples of poisons.

ARSENIC

Arsenic is a common element that is found in the Earth's crust (Figure 3.1) and has probably claimed more victims than any other poison. Elemental arsenic is a grey color and the salts are generally a white to yellow powder. Most arsenic compounds have no odor and have little or no taste and therefore can't be detected in food or water. Arsenic compounds make potent poisons. However, in today's modern toxicology laboratories, arsenic is easily detected.

Arsenic compounds have been used in insecticides, pesticides, herbicides, alloys, wood preservatives, additives to animal feed (some evidence suggests that small amounts of arsenic in the diet may be beneficial to animal growth and health), semiconductors and light-emitting diodes, homeopathic medicines, paints, and ceramics. As a poison, lewisite (an arsenic-containing gas) has been used militarily in chemical warfare. Intentional poisonings most often involve rodent poisons or pesticides containing arsenic. Accidental occupational exposure to arsenic compounds also occurs in industrial settings.

Arsenic compounds are primarily absorbed via the respiratory tract (inhaled) or orally. Once it is consumed, the majority (greater than 90%) of the arsenic is absorbed into the bloodstream, where it is then transported to the targets of its toxicity. The mechanism by which arsenic produces its effect is by combining chemically with sulfhydryl groups on proteins, such as enzymes, and thereby inactivating them.

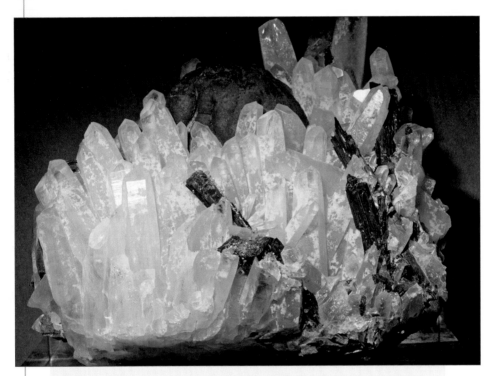

FIGURE 3.1   In this photograph taken in Peru, native dark-colored elemental arsenic is embedded in light-colored quartz crystals. Arsenic was commonly used in many murders until the arrival of the Marsh test, which detects the presence of this deadly poison.

Although arsenic is one of the oldest poisons used by humans, poisoning is less common today than in the past. However, they do still occur and sufficient doses of inorganic arsenic can result in death. Sublethal doses cause irritation of the stomach and intestines (stomach pain, nausea, vomiting, and diarrhea), anemia, arrhythmias (abnormal heart rhythm), sore throat and irritated lungs (if inhaled), impaired peripheral nerve function, and darkening of the skin, particularly on the palms and soles. The appearance of characteristic Mees lines, which are white lines in the finger- and toenails, develops several weeks following exposure.

Arsenic exposure has also been reported to increase the risk of cancer of the liver, bladder, kidneys, prostate, and lungs. Upon exposure, arsenic can be detected in blood, urine, gastric contents, and other tissues (including bone) by atomic absorption spectrophotometry. Arsenic can be measured in bone and hair for a long time after death, so the remains of many exhumed bodies have been studied to determine the role of arsenic in their deaths.

CYANIDE

Cyanide is a rapid-acting and deadly poison that can kill in a matter of minutes (Figure 3.2). Cyanide products are used in several industrial processes, including electroplating, metallurgy, and photographic processing. Cyanide is also a major byproduct of incomplete combustion and is frequently a component of toxic fire gases. Together with carbon monoxide, cyanide is an important cause of fire-related deaths. Hydrogen cyanide (HCN), also known as prussic acid or hydrocyanic acid, is used as a fumigant, for capital punishment in gas chambers, and for several other applications. It is a colorless, volatile liquid whose vapors can be inhaled and rapidly cause death. It is an agent that could also be used by terrorists as a chemical weapon.

Cyanide is found in salt forms such sodium cyanide and potassium cyanide. The salt forms are also very toxic and are often administered orally. Cyanide salts can also present an inhalation hazard when dissolved in acidic liquids. The salts of cyanide are strongly alkaline in solution and therefore corrosive to the digestive system when swallowed. Cyanide salts, which have a bitter taste and the odor of bitter almonds, are the common form used in intentional poisoning.

The toxicity of cyanide is due to its ability to stop cellular respiration and ATP (adenosine triphosphate, a source of cellular energy) synthesis in cells, causing what is called cytotoxic or metabolic **anoxia**. It deprives cells of the ability to use oxygen

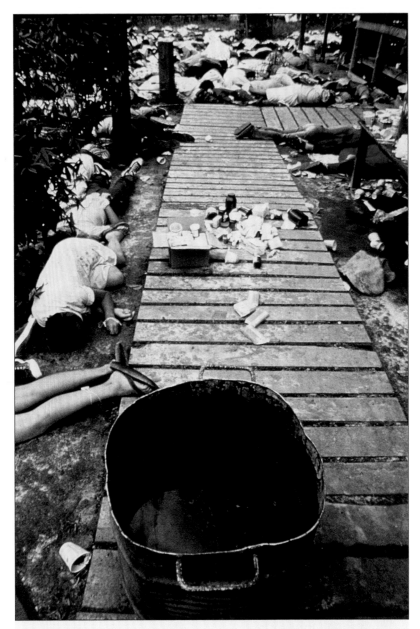

FIGURE 3.2 The bodies of cult members of the People's Temple, in Jonestown, Guyana, are strewn around a vat of a cyanide-laced drink. On November 18, 1978, cult leader Jim Jones ordered his followers to drink the poisonous mixture, which resulted in the deaths of 913 of his followers.

and thus has its strongest effects on tissues that have the greatest need for oxygen, namely, the brain and the heart. The symptoms of poisoning are relatively nonspecific and related to the cellular anoxia: headache, dizziness, nausea, vomiting, shortness of breath, and mental deterioration. Ultimately, seizures, coma, and cardiorespiratory collapse cause death.

STRYCHNINE

Strychnine is a colorless alkaloid obtained from the seeds of the *Strychnos nux-vomica* tree. It is extremely bitter with a highly detectable taste and it could only be hidden in foods and beverages that are also very bitter. It is used primarily for killing rodents. Fatal strychnine poisoning can occur following exposure via inhalation, oral administration, or absorption through the mucous membranes. Strychnine poisoning causes a violent and horrific death. It produces excruciatingly painful and violent spastic reactions that are commonly portrayed in the movies as the classic response to a poisoning. Following strychnine exposure, painful muscle cramps begin, which are followed by extremely intense muscle contractions that are worsened by the slightest external stimulus such as a simple touch. The convulsions appear to resemble seizures, but the victim is completely conscious and aware of the painful event. The contractions progress and eventually breathing is compromised and the person dies from asphyxiation. Rigor mortis sets in very rapidly and the deceased person is usually seen with an intense, blank, and frightening stare.

CARBON MONOXIDE

Carbon monoxide (CO) is a colorless, odorless, and tasteless gas produced by the incomplete combustion of organic materials. The most common sources of CO are faulty heating systems, automobile exhaust, fires, and cigarette smoke. CO produces its toxic effects by binding to hemoglobin in red blood cells and thus preventing oxygen from binding, which in turn causes tissue anoxia and impairment of ATP synthesis. The binding of CO to hemoglobin produces a molecule known as **carboxyhemoglobin**.

CO is the leading cause of accidental and intentional poisoning deaths in the United States. Like cyanide, the early symptoms of CO poisoning are relatively nonspecific and related to anoxia. These include progressively worsening headaches, nausea, fatigue, visual disturbances, mental confusion, and eventually coma and death. The symptoms of tissue hypoxia are similar to the flu and are often overlooked and not linked

Table 3.1 Deaths from Carbon Monoxide Poisoning in the United States, 1988–1996

YEAR	UNINTENTIONAL DEATHS	SUICIDES
1988	722	2,669
1989	756	2,212
1990	615	2,253
1991	614	2,208
1992	525	2,035
1993	549	2,068
1994	577	2,029
1995	533	2,071
1996	525	1,988
TOTAL	5,416	19,533

Source: U.S. Centers for Disease Control Data

to CO exposure. Prolonged exposure to CO can lead to brain damage and death.

CO is absorbed through the lungs and rapidly distributed to the red blood cells. CO binds to hemoglobin with 200 times greater affinity than oxygen. Carboxyhemoglobin saturation levels greater than 50% are usually fatal. Deaths have also occurred at lower levels in individuals who have preexisting health problems, such as heart disease, or who have other drugs present in them, such as alcohol. There is evidence that CO can inhibit cellular respiration, which contributes to its toxic or lethal effect. Most fire-related deaths are associated with abnormal carboxyhemoglobin levels. Lower levels would indicate that the person did not spend an extended period in the fire environment while they were alive; high levels indicate that the person survived for a more prolonged time. Very low carboxyhemoglobin levels (normal) could also indicate that the person died prior to the start of the fire. The most significant postmortem change in CO poisoning is a cherry red color of the blood, which manifests itself as a reddish coloration of the skin.

THALLIUM

Thallium is another metal found in the Earth's crust that has been used in the past as a rodent and ant poison and has been associated with poisoning deaths (Figure 3.3). It also has several industrial uses as well, such as in the manufacture of electronic devices, switches, the semiconductor industry, manufacture of special glass, and for certain medical procedures. Pure thallium has a bluish-white color and is a yellowish to white color when combined with other elements. Thallium sulfate is the form most commonly employed as a rat poison and it is odorless and tasteless. Its reputation as a human poison has lead to its banning in the United States

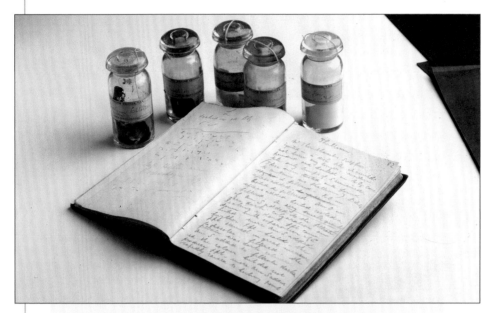

FIGURE 3.3 In 1861, chemist and physicist William Crookes discovered the element thallium. Crookes' thallium compounds and notebook detailing the discovery are displayed above.

because of safety issues. Thallium has not been produced in the United States since 1984.

Thallium has been used as an effective murder weapon. In most cases, exposure to thallium is likely to occur by mouth and it is almost completely absorbed following ingestion; occupational and accidental exposures can occur via inhalation. Following absorption, thallium distributes to the red blood cells and also appears in the brain, lung, gut, muscle tissue, salivary glands, pancreas, testes, spleen, kidney, liver, and bone. It can remain in the body for several weeks following exposure and with repeated doses will accumulate in the body over time.

Thallium is highly toxic due to its ability to mimic potassium in the body, which disrupts many cellular functions. Thallium is also a suspected cause of cancer. Characteristic symptoms of thallium poisoning include loss of hair, paresthesia (damage to peripheral nerves causing pain in the hands and feet described as a sensation of walking on hot coals), endocrine disorders, gastrointestinal and pulmonary distress, psychosis, delirium, and convulsions. Death may result from cardiorespiratory collapse. There is generally a delay before the onset of symptoms, which has contributed to its use as a homicidal poison.

ACONITE

Known by several colorful names such as wolf's bane, women's bane, monkshood, and devil's helmet, the *Aconitum napellus* plant (of the buttercup family) produces the poison aconite. All parts of the aconite plant are poisonous. Historically, aconite was used to poison arrow and lance tips, to kill condemned criminals, and to poison the water supply of enemies. It was once believed that aconite was the most toxic substance known to man.

Women were thought to be especially vulnerable to the poison. The Greek poet and physician Nicander of Colophon (second century B.C.) called aconite "woman-killer" and he said of aconite's toxicity: "It is established that of all poisons the quickest to act is aconite, and that death occurs on the same day if the genitals of a female are but touched by it." Reports of aconite poisoning continue to appear. Recently, toxicity has been seen with individuals using Chinese patent herbal medicines.

Aconite is a white powder that is soluble in alcohol and the poison targets the electrically excitable cells of the nervous, cardiovascular, and skeletal muscular tissues. Aconite can cause abnormal and potentially fatal heart rhythms. Aconite is a rapidly acting poison that takes effect within minutes of exposure. Early symptoms include a tingling and numbness at the point of contact, usually the mouth and throat. This sensation then spreads to the extremities and eventually the entire body is involved. Muscle weakness, visual and auditory disturbances, and convulsions precede death from respiratory failure.

RICIN

Ricin is a highly toxic protein extracted from the castor bean (Figure 3.4). Ricin comes from the waste products of castor oil production. It has been said that ricin is twice as deadly as cobra venom and it is poisonous if inhaled, injected, or ingested.

One of the major concerns is that, due to its availability and extreme toxicity, ricin is a potential weapon of terrorists. Al Qaeda is known to have shown interest in ricin as a bioterrorism agent and, in 2002, United States government officials asserted that the Islamic militant group, Ansar al-Islam, tested ricin, along with other chemical and biological agents, in northern Iraq. It is also suspected that ricin was used by the KGB, the Soviet secret police, during the Cold War for assassination. In a well-publicized incident in 1978, the Bulgarian Secret Service killed a dissident named Georgi Markov by injecting his leg with a small ricin-containing metallic pellet discharged from the tip of a modified umbrella. He became very ill and died a few days later. It is now known as the "umbrella murder."

Ricin's main effect is to inhibit protein synthesis in the body. According to the U.S. Centers for Disease Control, the following are the major symptoms of ricin poisoning, depending on the route of exposure. Following ingestion of ricin, the first symptoms usually occur in less than six hours.

- Inhalation: Difficulty breathing, fever, cough, nausea, and tightness in the chest. Heavy sweating may follow as well as fluid building up in the lungs. This would make breathing even more difficult, and the skin might turn blue; low blood pressure and respiratory failure may occur, eventually leading to death.

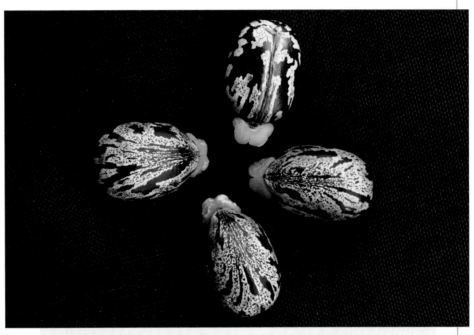

FIGURE 3.4 The toxic protein ricin is extracted from castor bean seeds. Ricin is highly poisonous. The extraction from only 1 or 2 seeds can kill a person.

- Ingestion: After ingesting ricin, the victim would develop vomiting and diarrhea that may become bloody. Severe dehydration may result, followed by low blood pressure. Other signs or symptoms may include hallucinations, seizures, and blood in the urine. Within several days, the person's liver, spleen, and kidneys might stop working, and the person could die.

- Skin and eye exposure: Ricin in the powder or mist form can cause redness and pain of the skin and the eyes.

Death takes place within 36 to 72 hours of exposure, depending on the route of exposure (inhalation, ingestion, or injection) and the dose received. If death has not occurred in 3 to 5 days, the victim usually recovers.

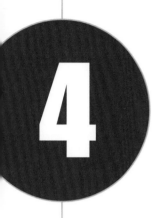

Poisoners in History

I would much prefer to suffer from the clean incision of an honest lancet than from a sweetened poison.

—Mark Twain (1835–1910)

Poisoning has been called the "coward's weapon" for its concealed approach to homicide. It has long been thought that poisoning is a favored method of females, but statistics do not support this notion, as many men have successfully practiced the art of poisoning throughout history. However, when women do commit murder, it's clear that poisoning is their first choice of weaponry.

Motive, intent, means, and opportunity are the ingredients of homicide, and poison certainly lends itself to the task at hand. The poisoner wishes to ensure that there are no witnesses and no visible signs of violence, since they hope to escape detection. The evolution of poisoners has its roots in the early history of humankind and the beginnings of civilization.

EARLY HISTORY OF POISONING

The Sumerians were the first to document the use of poisons and their effects. They were so enamored with poison they even worshiped a goddess of poisons, named Gula. Records of poisoning in Egypt date to 3000 B.C. and many plant- and animal-derived poisons have been used over the ages.

The early historical descriptions of poisoning are closely associated with mythology and a knowledge of poisons that rapidly developed in ancient times. For example, the Greeks were the first to use poison as a means of capital punishment—the Greek philosopher Socrates was executed by being made to drink poison (hemlock). In ancient Rome, poisoning was part of the dinner-time culture and became the most popular method for doing away with an unwanted rival. Poisoning became so much of a problem in the time of the Roman Empire that the Roman dictator Lucius Cornelius Sulla found it necessary to issue the world's first law against poisoning, called the Lex Cornelia in 82 B.C. Also, the emperor Trajan banned the growth of wolfsbane in Rome due to its popularity as a source of poison.

However, the incidences of poisoning continued to escalate at an alarming rate and continued to their peak in the first century. The roll call of Romans who were thought to be murdered by poison is too long to elaborate here.

The partial hit list includes Emperor Claudius (10 B.C. to A.D. 54), killed by his wife, Agrippina, so that her son Nero would assume the throne (Figure 4.1). Nero (A.D. 37–68), in turn, is known to have poisoned his brother, several wives, and many other untold rivals. He also unsuccessfully attempted to poison his mother after she became a threat to his power. The Roman emperors Vitellius, Domitian, Hadrian, Commodus, Caracalla, and Alexander Severus are all thought to have fallen victim to poison.

Similar events were also occurring in Asia and the East in early historical times. Writings indicate that the Chinese, Persians, and Indians were all developing their own expertise in poisons. In fact, the Indians were among the first to develop a secret service in the ancient world that used poison as a means of

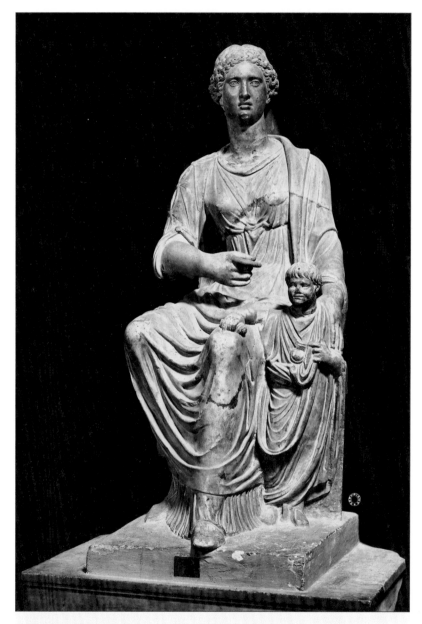

FIGURE 4.1 Agrippina the Younger sits beside her son Nero. According to legend, Agrippina killed her husband, Claudius, by serving him a plate of poisoned mushrooms in order for her son to assume the throne.

political assassination. *Visakanyas* ("poison damsels") were used to poison male targets by ingeniously taking advantage of the men's weakness for women. Frequently, poisons were concealed on a woman's body and delivered to the victim during amorous encounters. Alternatively, female poisoners won the trust of their victims by flirtatious means to gain the opportunity to blend poison into food or drink. Indians were also among the first, as early as 500 B.C., to write about the forensic detection of poisoners by examining their personality traits.

Two of the oldest existing works on the subject of poisons are *Theriaca* and *Alexipharmaca* by the Greek poet Nicander of Colophon (second century B.C.). *Theriaca* deals with the bites of venomous snakes, spiders, and scorpions, and how to remedy them. *Alexipharmaca* details further animal, vegetable, and mineral poisons, including aconite, white lead, hemlock, and opium, along with their symptoms and specific remedies. The treatment mostly includes herbal means and often olive oil as an emetic to induce vomiting. Similarly, in A.D. 40, Pedanius Dioscorides, a Greek physician and pharmacologist who practiced in Rome during the time of Nero, classified poisons and differentiated their origins in his five-volume discourse *Materia Medica*. This treatise was the authoritative textbook on the subject of poisons for centuries.

In 100 B.C., Mithradates VI, the king of Pontus (what is now Turkey), was considered to be a significant contributor to the idea of antidotes. He developed a universal antidote called Antidotum Mithridaticum, consisting of ingredients such as opium and honey. Every day, Mithridates VI took this antidote to thwart a possible poisoning. While the agents used would afford little protection based upon modern toxicological science, the idea of using chemical means to combat potential poisoning was instinctively accurate. It was his own fear of poisoning that led him to experiment with poisons and antidotes. Much of his experimentation was carried out on ill-fated criminals who were condemned to die. He even attempted to develop immunity by self-administering low levels of poisons every day. Ironically, upon the invasion of Pontus by Pompey the Great of Rome, Mithridates VI attempted suicide by taking poison, but he failed and needed to have a soldier stab him to death instead.

THE MIDDLE AGES AND RENAISSANCE

One of the major developments in the history of poisoning was the production of a powder form of arsenic, which is tasteless and odorless, making a perfect weapon of murder. It is often called the "poison of kings" or "inheritance powder." During the Middle Ages, arsenic became a popular choice as a poison and its availability became widespread.

As the Renaissance spread, so did the popularity of using poison as a means to do away with someone. Famous examples are found throughout the history of these times, but none as well known as the Borgia family (Figure 4.2). The name has forever been linked with the idea of a banquet full of toxic foods and beverages meant to put to death anyone who they no longer wished to walk this Earth. It is joked that no one ever claimed to have dined at Borgia's for dinner last night because no one survived to tell about the menu. The most notorious family member was Lucrezia Borgia: At extravagant parties thrown by the Borgia family, Lucrezia was in possession of a hollow ring that she used to poison drinks. Together with her brother Cesare and her father, the powerful Pope Alexander VI, they became legendary poisoners said to have murdered many political foes and probably a few of Lucrezia's lovers to boot.

By the late 1500s, poisoning reached almost epidemic proportions and spread throughout Europe. Poisoners and their potential victims shaped much of the historical record with

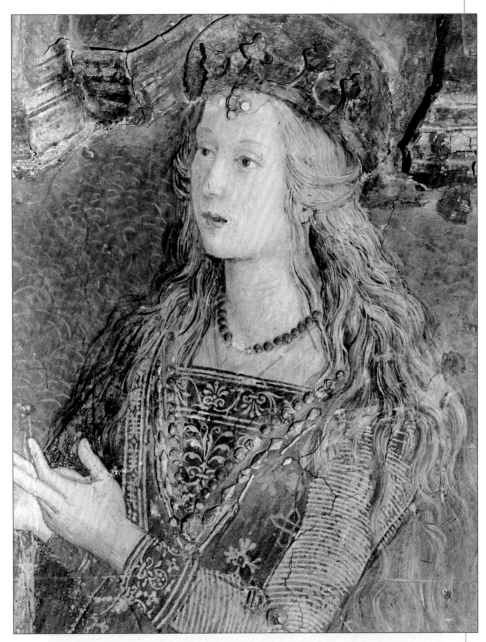

FIGURE 4.2 Lucrezia Borgia was the daughter of Pope Alexander VI. Lucrezia was rumored to be in possession of a hollow ring that she used to poison drinks of her family's enemies.

assassinations, murder, and the resultant paranoia. Tens of thousands of self-proclaimed and organized poisoners practiced their deadly trade. How-to textbooks were written by early chemists describing the proper ways of killing by poison and many were available for a fee to eliminate any and all potential rivals.

In Italy, schools of poisoning began to appear in the seventeenth century, which brought the murderous trade to a new level of sophistication, and secret poison societies were formed. Toxicology became an art form and experts were everywhere. Perhaps thousands of early earthly departures may be attributed to the skill of these lethal professionals (as well as dabbling amateurs). Sorcerers, magic spells, and the like were often nothing more than those that applied toxic chemicals to induce death and disease upon a sworn enemy.

An interesting example of mass poisoning (said to be responsible for more than 600 poisonings, including two popes) occurred when an arsenic-infused mixture called Acqua Toffana was invented by an Italian woman named Guilia Toffana. Acqua Toffana was sold as a ladies' cosmetic. While the concoction was marketed as a face makeup, female customers were told to speak with Madame Toffana to become skilled at the "other" use of the potion. Hundreds of wealthier widows appeared in Italy as a result of wearing the toxic makeup during encounters with unfortunate spouses. Eventually, the authorities caught up with Guilia Toffana and she was arrested, tortured, and strangled in prison in 1709.

LATER DEVELOPMENTS

By the seventeenth and eighteenth centuries, women had become even more entrenched in the art of poisoning. Secret societies, such as that developed by Hieronyma Spara, sprang up to teach women how to quietly kill their husbands. They received instructions on how to obtain poisons and then to administer them effectively. It was becoming public knowledge that one could commit murder by using the right poison.

It is thought that Catherine de Medici brought her understanding of poisons out of Italy and ultimately to France upon her marriage to King Henry II. She is credited with several murders in France, including a queen and a cardinal. Members of nobility throughout Europe became hysterical (with good reason), believing they were likely targets. Several attempts were made on the life of Queen Elizabeth I, such as a failed plot to smear an opium-based poison on her saddle pommel by a poisoner hired by Spain. Henry VIII was also reportedly targeted by a poisoner, and one successful murder was committed that involved the poisoning by arsenic of Marie Louise, wife of Carlos II of Spain, in 1689.

The practice of poisoning was not confined to Europe. George Washington was a target in 1776, when Thomas Hickey unsuccessfully attempted to assassinate him by feeding him poisoned peas. Hickey became the first American hanged for treason.

Poisoning became so prevalent that naturally occurring diseases were often misdiagnosed as a poisoning. Due to their paranoia, many nobles would not eat any food that was prepared by others, or else they acquired food tasters as a necessary precaution. Priests were inundated with confessions of poisoning, as individuals who knew they could get away with murder in this life became concerned with the consequences of their actions in the hereafter. Eventually, an attempt to limit the sale of poison was made and investigations of homicide by poisoning became more commonplace. However, one can imagine that few culprits were actually apprehended and charged. Interestingly, the investigations did nothing but draw attention to the subject of poisons, so that even more people learned how to use them.

While poisoning for personal gain is found throughout the ages, many believe that the glory days of poisoners were in the Victorian era in the nineteenth century. One of the most famous cases involved Napoleon, who was alleged to have been a victim of arsenic poisoning. When Napoleon became ill in 1820, he was certain that he was being poisoned by a growing conspiracy. However, popular belief holds that it was moldy wallpaper that may have released a poisonous gas, or perhaps medicines that he was consuming, that contributed to Napoleon's illness.

By the nineteenth century, poisoning was no longer a trade practiced exclusively by and against nobility—it was readily available to anyone with a motive. Now, poison for profit had a new lure: life insurance. Poison for profit was at an all-time high and no one could be certain how many fell victim to these acts and were simply buried with their secret.

Table 4.1 Poisoner's Background

GROUP	% OF CASES
General public	71
Physician	8
Political figure	4
Nurse	4
Other	5
Unknown	9

Source: Trestrail, John Harris. *Criminal Poisoning: Investigational Guide for Law Enforcement, Toxicologists, Forensic Scientists and Attorneys.* Totowa, NJ: Humana Press, 2000.

Laws were needed to bring things under control. For example, the Arsenic Act of 1851 was directed at decreasing the frequency of poisoning. It was also during this period that a new field was born out of the need to stem the tide of poisonings: forensic toxicology. The challenge to scientists to develop sensitive and accurate methods for detection of poisons at this time became the basis for modern toxicological practices. Pioneers like Marsh and Riensch developed methods for the detection of some of the common poisons of the time, such as arsenic, and new scientific weapons against the poisoners were starting to lead to more convictions.

POISONING IN THE PRESENT DAY

Physicians with gambling problems, husbands with mistresses, serial killers, jealous husbands, relatives looking for financial gains, poisoning neighbors, product tampering, and political assassins: The list of modern day poisoners and their motives seems endless, and examples of poisoning are continuing to be exposed today. It isn't just about eliminating the unwanted family members or rivals anymore. Governments and terrorists have been carrying out research into the possibility of using poisons as weapons.

On the other hand, the growth of the field of toxicology has made most poisons easily detectable today. The poisoner has a much more difficult time with respect to the poison not being detected. It must, however, be emphasized that even some readily detectable poisons may not be always found using routine screening methods. There are no catchall procedures in forensic toxicology (contrary to what's shown frequently on TV). In many cases, a lack of suspicion of a possible poisoning can result in a failure to detect a drug or poison. The importance of a proper investigation of the scene and circumstances of a death, and of cooperation between investigators and forensic scientists, is crucial to uncovering such crimes.

Sadly, the drug culture that flourished in the twentieth century, and continues to expand today, is now the greatest contributor to the loss of life by chemical means. Legal drugs used to save lives, as well as numerous illegal drugs, have now been added to the list of poisons that the toxicologist must contend with. Cocaine, heroin, amphetamines, insulin, muscle relaxants, barbiturates, and environmental and occupation chemicals have joined carbon monoxide, arsenic, and cyanide as possible sources of overdose and poisoning. Common household and industrial chemicals such as paints, gasoline, glues, or any number of other chemicals are potentially lethal to a small child or a suicidal adult, but are also known for their abuse potential. Sometimes the poisoner is one and same as the victim.

FAMOUS POISONINGS IN HISTORY

Throughout history, there have been a number of famous poisonings and poisoners that have captured the attention of the general public. Poisoners have often been given memorable nicknames by the media, and the trials of infamous poisoners inevitably draw swarms of reporters eager to provide shocking details of the crime. What follows are short biographical sketches of some of the most notorious poisoners to date.

Claudius and Agrippina

The Roman emperor Claudius was poisoned by his wife Empress Agrippina. She was a cunning woman who poisoned her husband's mushrooms so that she could have the throne to herself until her son Nero was old enough to take over. Nero later commented on how mushrooms were "the food of the gods," proving he knew of the murder plot devised by his mother. Agrippina is also believed to have arranged the deaths of several others.

Nannie Doss

Nannie Doss was known by the name Arsenic Annie because she killed 11 family members with this favored poison. She was born in 1905 with the original name Nancy Hazle, and she earned the nickname The Giggling Granny because she always seemed to be laughing and smiling, even after her eventual arrest. Unsuspecting victims were fed prunes (Granny's healthy favorite) laced with rat poison. She is thought to have killed her two daughters (originally thought to have died from food poisoning), her mother, mother-in-law, and several other unlucky family members and acquaintances. Arsenic Annie was married several times and at least four of her husbands met with untimely deaths. Finally, following the death of her last husband, Samuel Doss, she was found guilty of murder.

Dr. Edward Pritchard

The last public execution in Scotland was that of an infamous doctor, Edward Pritchard, found guilty of poisoning his wife and mother-in-law. Pritchard was an adulterous surgeon who performed an abortion on his servant girl after she became pregnant with his child. In November 1864, his wife became very ill. When her mother came to care for her, she also began to show symptoms of a mysterious illness. By February 1865, Pritchard's mother-in-law died and only a month later his wife also passed away. It was not until the authorities received an anonymous letter that the bodies were exhumed and the cause of death was determined to be antimony poisoning. Dr. Pritchard was convicted of these murders and then executed in front of more than 100,000 spectators.

Mary Ann Cotton

She's dead and she's rotten.

She lies in her bed

With her eyes wide open.

Sing, sing!

"Oh, what can I sing?

Mary Ann Cotton is

tied up with string."

Where, where?

"Up in the air—selling

black puddings a

penny a pair."

Born Mary Ann Robson in 1832, this female poisoner became the subject of a popular English children's rhyme. Mary Ann Cotton had a very difficult childhood in the nineteenth century. When she grew up, she was determined never to find herself poor and on the streets again. Her killing streak began and ended only after she had killed 3 of her husbands, 10 of her children (mostly infants), her own mother and sister, 5 of her stepchildren, and a man named Nattrass. All of her victims mysteriously came down with gastric fever and various other intestinal disorders.

Cotton was able to murder so many because after the death of each of her family members and the collection of insurance money (perhaps motivated by her desire never to be poor again), she would move on. Using this method, she was never in one place long enough for the neighbors and doctors to become suspicious. Finally, after the death of her son Charles people caught on and she received so much publicity that her next husband (and likely victim) was scared off. She was arrested, found guilty, and during her hanging she struggled for three minutes (due to improper execution procedure), ending her life with a slow, agonizing death.

Velma Barfield

Velma Barfield was an infamous American serial poisoner. She was placed on death row after poisoning her latest husband, Stuart Taylor. One of the more disturbing aspects of Velma Barfield was her image as a sweet, Christian grandmother who nursed her sickly victims until they died of arsenic poisoning. After being caught, she stood by her claim that she was only trying to make her husband sick and did not think he would die. Unfortunately for her, this was not the best defense approach, due to the fact that many previous victims, including her mother, elderly employers, and other family

Table 4.2
Most Common Poisons Used by Poisoners

POISON	% OF CASES
Arsenic	31
Cyanide	9
Strychnine	6
Morphine	3
Chloroform	2
All other poisons	50

Source: Trestrail, John Harris. *Criminal Poisoning: Investigational Guide for Law Enforcement, Toxicologists, Forensic Scientists and Attorneys.* Totowa, NJ: Humana Press, 2000.

members, died from strikingly similar diseases. The prosecution wanted to know why she did not come forward when her victim's case worsened so the antidote could be administered. This also weakened her defense. Barfield's lawyers argued that the prescription drugs to which she was addicted hindered her judgment, and this was confirmed by her physicians. In the end, her lawyer made the mistake of putting her on the stand, where she made some rather disturbing remarks to the prosecution's questioning, indicating that she did not feel personally responsible for their deaths.

Barfield was convicted of first-degree murder and sent to jail awaiting execution. She immediately experienced powerful **withdrawal** symptoms due to the unavailability of her prescription drugs. She then declared herself a born-again Christian and did acts of kindness around the jail and maintained contact with famous evangelical Christian Billy Graham. This, however, failed to change the outcome of her appeal and on November 2, 1984, she became the first woman put to death by lethal injection in the United States.

Dr. Hawley Harvey Crippen

In 1910, Dr. Hawley Harvey Crippen became known as the first criminal to be caught by wireless communication as he was fleeing England aboard the U.S.S. *Montrose*. This American homeopathic doctor poisoned his wife, Belle Elmore, with **hyoscine** after a party and began carefully disposing of the body parts (some parts were placed in the tub and dissolved while others were put in the oven). Those who knew him became suspicious when his secretary, Ethel Le Neve, moved in immediately after his wife's death and began wearing Belle's clothing and jewelry. Crippen was questioned by Chief Inspector Dew and he was presumed innocent despite changing his story multiple times.

Crippen, however, became nervous and fled with Le Neve. This aroused the suspicions of Inspector Dew, who found human remains in Dr. Crippen's basement. While aboard the *Montrose* and headed for Canada, Crippen was recognized, even though he was using a fake name and had shaved his moustache; Le Neve was disguised as his son. The ship used its radio to contact the authorities. Inspector Dew boarded a much faster ship and was waiting for Crippen when he arrived in Canada. Dew boarded the ship disguised as a pilot and surprised Crippen and Le Neve. Both were taken back to England

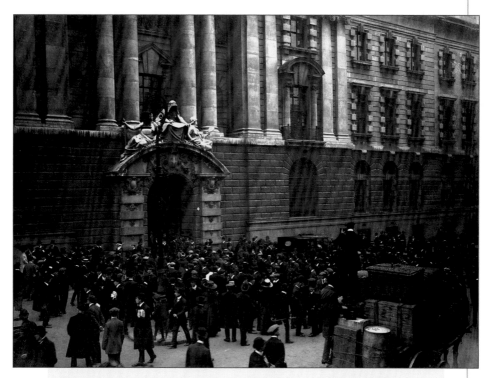

FIGURE 4.3   The above photograph was taken in August 1910, outside the Old Bailey law court during the trial of Dr. Hawley Harvey Crippen. Dr. Crippen was found guilty and sentenced to death for poisoning his wife with hyoscine.

and put on trial, but only Crippen was convicted of murder (Figure 4.3). He was hanged on November 23, 1910. In England, the word *Crippen* is still used as a synonym for poisoner.

The Mensa Murderer

George Trepal, also known as the Mensa Murderer because he was a member of the high I.Q society Mensa, committed the almost perfect crime. Trepal lived in Florida and had noisy neighbors. For years, he yelled at the Carrs to turn their music down. Then suddenly, all the members of the Carr family began to come down with a mysterious illness. The mother, Peggy Carr, died, leaving everyone confused over the cause of her disease, while other members of the family were in critical condition. The doctors ultimately determined the cause to be thallium poisoning.

Their house was searched carefully and residue of thallium salt was found in Coke bottles (Figure 4.4). The subsequent investigation ultimately led to their neighbor, George Trepal. An FBI search of Trepal's house found chemistry books and equipment, poison information, and a bottle-capping machine (which could put caps back on soda bottles after poison had been added). They also found a copy of the novel *Pale Horse* by Agatha Christie, a story in which a family is poisoned by thallium. The murderous genius was tried and sentenced to death.

Stella Nickell

Stella Nickell was convicted of killing her husband, Bruce, and Sue Snow by tampering with Excedrin, a common over-the-counter pain reliever. Both Bruce and Sue died of cyanide poisoning in 1986 and it was at first believed that there was some member of the public that was poisoning Excedrin products and placing them back on drugstore and/or supermarket shelves. Sue Snow was thought to be one of the unlucky victims who had purchased a contaminated product.

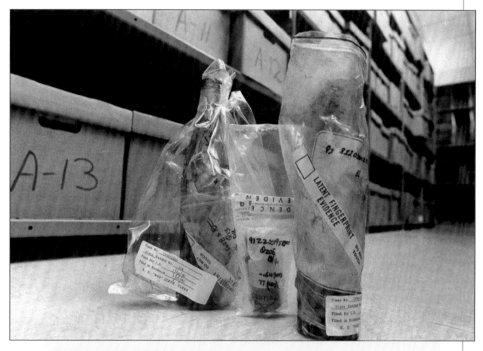

FIGURE 4.4 Coca-Cola bottles tainted with thallium served as evidence against murderer George Trepal, who fatally poisoned his neighbor, Peggy Carr. Trepal laced his neighbor's drinks because he believed that she and her family were too loud.

Tests found particles of algae killer (for use in fish tanks) in the tainted products. Stella owned a fish tank but said that she never purchased algae killer. The owner of a local pet store, however, told authorities that she bought so much algae killer that he had to order it specially for her. Stella's daughter, Cindy Hamilton, came forward and testified that her mother went to the library to research poisons and had talked about killing her husband. Stella was sentenced to 90 years in prison. Today, some people believe that Stella was wrongfully imprisoned and seek to prove her innocence, claiming that those who testified against her received large sums of money.

Jim Jones

Jim Jones was responsible for the mass poisoning of the cult-like religious community in Guyana that he had established. He began the People's Temple church and had gained nearly 1,000 followers by the 1950s. Many praised him for his ability to establish a church that provided equal treatment of its African-American and impoverished members. Jones's views began to diverge from mainstream Christianity and border on socialism; Jones also proclaimed himself messiah. When his group's practices were investigated by the U.S. government, Jones moved the People's Temple to Jonestown, Guyana (a city named after him). Jones was also addicted to drugs (including marijuana and LSD), which he could no longer hide from the members of his organization.

In November 1978, United States Representative Leo Ryan traveled to Jonestown to investigate this closed community. Although the beginning of the trip went well, Ryan discovered about 20 people who wished to leave the community. After an attempt on the life of the representative, the group hurried to the airstrip to leave. A group of armed guards arrived before they boarded the plane and Ryan, members of the news crew, and a member of the People's Temple who was fleeing with them were killed. The rest managed to escape. Later that day, the 913 remaining members of the People's Temple committed suicide (an act they had planned and simulated for years in advance), under the orders of Jones, by drinking a fruit drink laced with cyanide. Jones was later found dead of a gunshot wound. It is believed that Jones had convinced his followers that they would go with him to another planet to live and the only way to achieve this goal was mass suicide.

Genene Jones

Genene Jones was a nurse who joined the ranks of the Angels of Death, infamous caregivers who kill their patients. What makes the case of Genene Jones stand out is that her targets were infants and young children who could not tell others what she was doing to them. She started her career as a nurse in Bexar County Medical Center Hospital. When the first child she cared for died, she started sobbing and consoling the parents. This excitement and attention was just what she was seeking.

Doctors and other nurses became suspicious of the high number of cardiac arrests and seizures that were occurring while Jones was on duty. Her coworkers called her shift the "death shift" because so many children died on it, many more than on any other shift. When she was not present, the children would make dramatic improvements. Many of the deaths were attributed to overdoses of heparin, an anti-blood clotting drug.

Jones was also thought to suffer from Munchausen syndrome, a psychological disorder characterized by constantly faking illness to gain attention. It was thought that this syndrome also caused her to create illness in others, which brought the attention upon her while she cared for them.

Jones moved to a clinic opened by Dr. Holland, a former coworker, after all nurses were fired from the hospital ward because of the mysterious deaths. Then, Dr. Holland's clinic began experiencing a string of unexplained deaths due to succinylcholine overdoses, a muscle relaxant that puts patients in a helpless state of paralysis.

There was now enough evidence to convict Jones. She was sentenced to life in prison for the murder of one child patient and for intentionally harming another. Jones is believed to have murdered nearly 50 infants and harmed many others who managed to escape with their lives.

Charles Cullen

More recently, a nurse named Charles Cullen admitted to poisoning dozens of sick patients in hospitals in New Jersey (Figure 4.5). He used insulin, a **hormone** that is used to control blood sugar levels but which in overdose can produce fatal hypoglycemia. In some cases he used digoxin, a drug used to treat abnormal heart rhythms, but which is toxic in high doses. At the time of these revelations his victims had already been embalmed and buried.

This type of case presents many challenges for the forensic toxicologist, some of which cannot be satisfactorily resolved. Insulin levels are only tested in blood samples, but not in tissues, in an unembalmed body; hence forensic toxicology cannot be performed on samples taken from exhumed bodies even

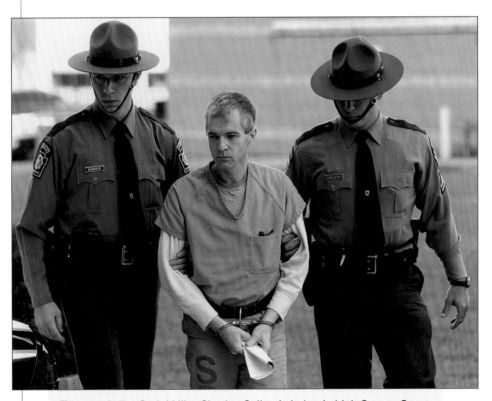

FIGURE 4.5 Serial killer Charles Cullen is led to Lehigh County Court in Allentown, PA, November 17, 2004. Cullen admitted to killing more than 40 people from poisonous injections, during his time working as a nurse. Cullen was sentenced to 11 consecutive life sentences.

where insulin overdosing is involved. Digoxin can be detected in exhumed bodies but the results may not always be readily interpreted. If the patient was not being prescribed digoxin, then the qualitative detection of the drug would confirm this detail of the confession. However, if the patient was being prescribed digoxin, extreme care must be exercised in interpreting the quantitative results in embalmed/exhumed victims. Factors that can cause drug level changes in buried bodies must be carefully considered and evaluated. Low levels may not always reflect the absence of an overdose before death. On the other hand, very high levels may cautiously be considered as consistent with poisoning. Finally, it may be noted that the increase in dosage of a prescribed drug in a seriously ill patient is perhaps the most diabolical example of homicidal poisoning and poses one of the most difficult challenges in case interpretation to the forensic toxicologist.

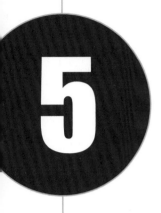

Drugs of Abuse

Drugs are generally not labeled as poisons, but they have been used as poisons for centuries. Even though all drugs are toxic at high doses, a poison is defined as a chemical agent for which there is no known therapeutic use. With that said, at high doses drugs pass from being therapeutic to toxic. There are many drugs that have a high abuse potential and these contribute significantly to health, economic, and personal problems.

Morphine tops the list of drugs that are used as poisons, although drugs and alcohol seem to be involved in all types of crimes. Some drugs of abuse have **psychoactive** properties and target mainly the **central nervous system (CNS).** Others also target the CNS but are not considered psychoactive, such as narcotics. Performance-enhancing drugs, such as **anabolic steroids**, are also abused but they do not target the CNS.

Drug users are more likely to commit violent crimes, be involved in accidents, lose their jobs, be placed in severe financial hardship, and die at a younger age, either directly or indirectly as a result of drug use. Unfortunately, drug abuse is not a victimless crime and the population at large is also at risk. Recreational drug use is widespread and certain populations, especially the young, are likely to use psychoactive agents. As many as 34% of college students in the United States have used illicit drugs, with marijuana being the most common drug followed by cocaine, amphetamines, heroin and other opiate drugs, inhalants, **tranquilizers**, and hallucinogens. Of course,

Table 5.1 Drugs with Abuse Potential

DRUG	EXAMPLES
CNS Depressants	
Ethanol	All alcoholic beverages
Benzodiazepines	Alprazolam, diazepam, flunitrazepam, oxazepam, temazepam, triazolam
Opiates	Morphine, heroin, codeine, fentanyl, methadone, oxycodone, meperidine
Marijuana	Tetrahydrocannabinol (THC)
Barbiturates	Phenobarbital, secobarbital, thiopental
CNS Stimulants	
Cocaine	Crack, free base, cocaine (HCL)
Amphetamines	Amphetamine, methamphetamine, methylenedioxymethamphetamine (MDMA), methyldioyamphetamine (MDA)
Other Psychoactive Classes	
Hallucinogens	LSD, psilocybin, mescaline
Dissociative anesthetics	PCP, ketamine, dextromethorphan
Inhalants	Volatile solvents, aerosols, gases, propellants

the legal use of alcohol still outpaces all the others. Alcohol use is frequently associated with car accidents, homicides, drug deaths, date rapes, and suicides. Opiates and cocaine predominate as contributors to direct drug-related deaths. Other drugs such as amphetamines and marijuana are often associated with nondrug overdose deaths.

ALCOHOL (ETHANOL)

Ethanol (CH_3CH_2OH) is probably one of the oldest drugs used by humans and it remains the most commonly consumed drug in most Western societies. More than 80% of the world's adult population uses some form of alcohol in varying amounts. Of those, some 10% regularly use alcohol to the extent that it constitutes abusive behavior. The mortality rate is 50% higher in persons consuming six or more drinks per day as compared to nondrinkers. Alcohol contributes to deaths in a variety of ways, including violent crimes, suicides, accidental deaths, child abuse, and drug-related deaths.

Ethanol is a product of fermentation by the action of yeast cells on sugars found in fruits and grains. The content of alcoholic beverages varies for different types of drinks. Ethanol is a clear, volatile liquid that is soluble in water and has a characteristic taste and odor. As a drug, ethanol falls into the category of a **central nervous system (CNS) depressant** with the predominant effect of depressing brain function.

CNS depression is directly linked to a person's blood alcohol concentration (BAC): As BAC rises, so does the degree of CNS depression. The American Medical Association has defined the blood alcohol concentration where impairment begins to be 0.04% (grams of ethanol per 100 milliliters of blood). In most of the United States, a person is legally intoxicated at a BAC of 0.08% and considered to be impaired at 0.05%.

Once ethanol is absorbed, it moves throughout the body via the blood into other tissues. It is distributed to the body water and the greater the water contents of a tissue, the greater the distribution of ethanol to that tissue (e.g., brain tissue has a greater ETOH concentration than bone tissue). The factors that determine BAC are the volume of alcohol consumed, whether consumption was with or without food, body weight, gender, and distribution (based on the total body water) of ethanol.

Because men and women have different body water amounts—men average 68% and women 55%—there are differences between the ethanol concentration in men and women of similar weight after consuming alcohol. In other words, if a man and a woman of the same weight drink equivalent amounts of alcohol, the woman will have a higher BAC. Similarly, if two men of different body weights drink the same amount of alcohol, the lighter man will have a higher BAC. In general, the less you weigh the more you will be affected by a given amount of alcohol.

Another important factor that will affect the BAC is the rate at which ethanol is eliminated. BAC is a function of the balance between how much is entering the blood versus how much is cleared or removed. Most of the ethanol is removed by the liver via metabolism, with lesser amounts excreted in the breath, urine, feces, perspiration, and saliva. The rate at which ethanol is cleared from the blood varies from one individual to another. Heavy drinkers and alcoholics tend to eliminate alcohol much faster than the inexperienced drinker. In most individuals, the rate of alcohol clearance from blood ranges from 0.01% to 0.025% per hour, with an average of 0.017%.

This is very important for the forensic toxicologist. For example, say an accident occurs at midnight and the alcohol content of blood from the driver at the hospital two hours later was 0.07%. Does this mean that the level was below 0.08% at the time

Table 5.2 Alcohol Content of Various Beverages

BEVERAGE	ALCOHOL CONTENT (%)
Beer (lager)	3.2–4.5
Table wine	7.1–14.0
Sparkling wine	8.0–14.0
Brandy	40.0–43.0
Whisky	40.0–75.0
Vodka	40.0–50.0
Gin	40.0–48.5
Tequila	45.0–50.5

of the accident? Not necessarily. Let's assume that the person stopped drinking prior to the accident so that all the ethanol was absorbed from the person's gastrointestinal tract at midnight. We can calculate the BAC to the time of the accident by using the average clearance rate of 0.017% per hour for two hours: The BAC two hours earlier would be 0.104% (legally intoxicated).

So, what happens when a person starts to drink alcohol? At first, as the BAC begins to rise and there is an apparent stimulatory effect, the person may become more talkative or loud. They may seem more social and have increased self-confidence. This is not a stimulatory effect but rather a depression of inhibitory centers of the brain. As the BAC increases, impairment of judgment, decision making, perception, motor function, and reaction time occurs. Significant and progressive reduction in mental and physical abilities continues as BAC rises and the person is visibly intoxicated. A BAC over 0.30% can result in loss of consciousness and possible death; with concentrations over 0.40%, death becomes increasingly likely. Chronic, heavy use of alcohol leads to a high incidence of brain damage; liver disease; heart disease; stroke; metabolic disorders; and oral, lung, and liver cancers, and abuse during pregnancy also increases the risk of fetal malformations.

Tolerance is the lessening of the effectiveness of a drug after a period of prolonged or heavy use. Studies have shown that chronic alcohol users can have at least twice the tolerance for alcohol as an average person. It is important to note that even in heavy alcohol users, impairment is clearly measurable at the blood alcohol concentration levels that are currently used for traffic law enforcement. However, even with cognitive impairment, many highly tolerant individuals are capable of engaging in physical activities and actions (including fighting) at levels that would result in unconsciousness or even death in nontolerant individuals.

COCAINE

Cocaine is a strongly addictive **stimulant** that has its effect on the brain. Cocaine has become an extremely popular abused drug during the last few decades and forensic cases involving cocaine are commonplace. However, cocaine is not a new drug— it has been used in some form for thousands of years. Cocaine is derived from the leaf of the *Erythroxylon coca* bush, which grows primarily in the Andean mountains in South America. At one time, it was popular to find cocaine in many fashionable "miracle" tonics and elixirs said to cure many ailments. It was even found at one time in the popular soft drink Coca-Cola. Memorable advertising slogans such as "delicious and refreshing for headache and exhaustion"; "the favorite drink for ladies when thirsty, weary, and despondent"; "revives and sustains"; "full of vim, vigor and go" all appear to reflect the stimulant nature of the product.

Cocaine is a Schedule II drug, meaning that it has some medicinal value but also a high potential for abuse. There are two common forms of cocaine on the illicit drug market: the white crystalline powder, which is commonly used by snorting (intra-nasally) or injecting intravenously, and crack cocaine, the form of cocaine that is smoked. Pure cocaine is often cut with substances such as cornstarch, talcum powder, or sugar, or with active drugs such as caffeine, codeine, procaine, or amphetamines.

Cocaine is a serious problem in the United States: An esti-mated 500,000 people are current crack users and three to four times that number are addicted to, or regularly abusing, all forms of cocaine. Smoking crack cocaine, the user experiences very powerful and rapid onset of effects. Crack is an inexpensive drug that is very popular with less affluent drug abusers, while cocaine powder is more commonly used by middle- and upper-class drug abusers. The age group with the greatest current use is 18 to 25 years old. Men seem to use the drug more than women. The primary routes of exposure for cocaine are intra-nasal (snorting), inhalation (smoking), intravenous (injecting), and oral (chewing). Injecting cocaine produces the most rapid effects (almost immediate).

The regions of the brain most affected by cocaine are involved with the reward centers, a key in basic pleasurable stimuli such as sex, food, and water intake. Cocaine prevents the reuptake of a neurotransmitter called **dopamine** involved in many of these functions (Figure 5.1). When pleasurable events take place, a large amount of dopamine is released in the brain. Normally, the dopamine is then removed as it is pumped back into the neurons from which it was released and the reward signal is stopped. Cocaine prevents the dopamine from being removed

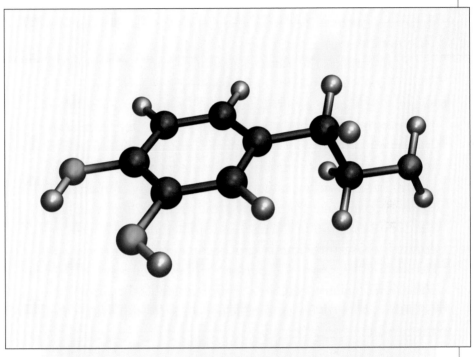

FIGURE 5.1   In this computer model of a dopamine molecule, the different atoms are color-coded: carbon *(red)*, hydrogen *(white)*, oxygen *(green)*, and nitrogen *(orange)*. Dopamine has many functions within the brain, but it is most commonly associated with feelings of pleasure induced by food, sex, or drugs.

and prolongs these effects in the brain, continuing to stimulate the reward centers. The buildup of dopamine is associated with the **euphoria** that develops.

The adverse effects of cocaine include cardiovascular complications, psychosocial problems, and **addiction**. Like other drugs, cocaine abuse can lead to tolerance and the drug abuser requires more and more drug to produce the desired effect. Powerful cravings develop and the person seeks more of the drug. Ultimately, in most chronic users, the cravings exceed the ability of the user to take sufficient drug, and dangerous psychological and behavioral patterns develop. Severe psychosis is a result in most chronic abusers.

Cocaine makes the user feel euphoric, stimulated, and alert. The person may have difficulty sleeping and experience a loss of appetite. Cocaine causes increases in heart rate and blood pressure and causes body temperature to rise. One forensically important unfavorable outcome is cocaine-induced excited delirium, a group of symptoms associated with cocaine intoxication that include hyperthermia (elevated body temperature), delirium, paranoia, abnormally great strength, highly agitated state, cardiorespiratory arrest, and sudden death. When confronted, these individuals can become very aggressive and defiant and users often experience episodes of psychotic and sometimes violent behavior. Unfortunately, they often die while in custody of law enforcement during attempts to restrain the person.

Another important forensic example of cocaine toxicity is death due to body packing. Body packing is the practice of transporting drugs by swallowing or vaginally or rectally inserting the drug within the body in a condom, balloon, or other containment device. Sometimes these containers burst, releasing the contents into the body resulting in a massive overdose. Blood cocaine levels are usually very high making interpretation of these results relatively clear-cut.

The drug most commonly used in combination with cocaine is alcohol. There is a potentially dangerous drug interaction between ethanol and cocaine. When taken at the same time, they are converted to a chemical known as **cocaethylene** by the body. The effects last longer with cocaethylene and it is more toxic than either drug alone. Deaths resulting from the consumption of these two drugs is much higher when they are used in combination.

OPIATES

Opiates obtained from the opium poppy (*Papaver somniferum*) have been used for more than 2,000 years (Figure 5.2). Morphine is an **opioid** drug and has been a common poison over the decades. The drugs in this family are chemically related to morphine or a derivative of morphine and they are all addictive and potentially deadly.

The action of these drugs is based on compounds produced by the body called endorphins, enkephalins, and dynorphins, which act as natural painkillers. The opiate drugs work through

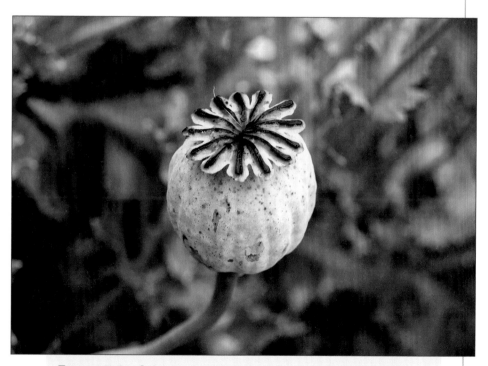

FIGURE 5.2 Opium, a narcotic drug, is extracted from the opium poppy (*Papaver somniferum*), seen above.

the same pathway in the body, binding to the same receptors in the brain. These drugs are potent narcotic **analgesic** (pain-killing) drugs and strong cough suppressants. Side effects include mental clouding, euphoria, drowsiness, and visual disturbances. Opiates also have an anorexic effect (decreases hunger) and they produce constipation.

Morphine and other related opiates are highly addictive and subject to tolerance. The psychological and **physical dependence** develops quickly and users become quite ill from withdrawal if the drug is unavailable. At high doses, they cause potentially fatal **respiratory depression**. There are more than 30 opiate drugs available today, including codeine, dihydrocodeine, fentanyl, hydrocodone, methadone, pentazocine, propoxyphene, oxyco-done, oxymorphone, and heroin. Of these, the most abused and most often fatal is heroin.

Heroin is an illegal derivative of morphine that is produced in clandestine laboratories. It is a Schedule I drug, meaning that it has no medical use and a high potential for abuse. It is the most abused opiate drug and it is typically found as a white powder mixed with sugars or as a black sticky sub-stance called "black tar." The heroin available today is more pure than in times past but is still often cut before it reaches the street. Therefore, the strength of the heroin can vary greatly, making it difficult for the user to gauge the risk of fatal overdose.

More than 3.5 million people in the United States have tried heroin and more than 200,000 are dependent on the drug. Heroin use has remained stable over the last few years and the number of emergency overdose cases has also not changed. The most common route of exposure for heroin has classically been intravenous injection, but it is also snorted or smoked, methods that are more popular among younger users. The greater purity of heroin today makes inhalation methods more likely, which has opened up the heroin market to abusers who have an aversion to injecting drugs. Also, users tend to mistakenly believe that sniffing or smoking heroin will not lead to addiction.

From the blood, heroin rapidly enters the brain, where it exerts its effects. Heroin is quickly converted to morphine and other metabolites. Heroin is more fat-soluble than morphine, so it enters the brain faster, causing a more intense rush that is particularly addictive. Other side effects of heroin include severe itching, flushing, dry mouth, nausea, and vomiting.

Fentanyl is a synthetic narcotic painreliever that is extremely fast-acting. It is 50 to 100 times more potent than morphine and abusers who overdose have been found dead with the needle

Body Packers

Sometimes people will ingest drugs to hide the evidence when confronted by law authorities. As police close in, people panic and swallow the drug rather than face possible arrest. Unfortunately, they often overdose and toxicity ensues. The effects are usually more severe than recreational drug overdose because of the large doses. In related cases, individuals ingest drugs as a means of transporting or smuggling drugs across borders. Body packers, as they are called, transport large quantities of drug by carefully packaging the drug in what is believed to be secure and less likely to rupture materials (balloons, condoms, etc.). They consume the packages by either swallowing them or inserting them into a body cavity. Individuals have suffered fatal overdoses when the packaging breaks, causing the drug to be released and absorbed into the bloodstream.

still in their arm. Because of its high fat solubility, fentanyl is available in transdermal patches that slowly release the drug into the bloodstream for treatment of chronic pain. Other members of the fentanyl class used therapeutically are alfentanyl and sufentanyl, the latter much more potent than fentanyl itself. Alpha-methyl fentanyl (designer drug fentanyl) is the most potent form and its use even in very small amounts can produce coma and death.

MARIJUANA

Cannabinoids (marijuana) are not associated with fatalities due to overdose. The active component in marijuana is **delta 9-tetrahydrocannabinol** (THC). There are no reports of individuals dying from THC alone, but THC is detected in a fairly significant number of deaths, particularly those due to overdose of other drugs and violent or accidental deaths.

The two routes of exposure to marijuana are smoking or oral ingestion. THC enters the brain fairly rapidly and the effects last from about one to three hours. If marijuana is ingested, the effects take longer to occur but they tend to last longer as well. Smoking marijuana delivers more drug than oral consumption and the effect (high) tends to be more intense. THC causes an increased heart rate, dilation of the blood vessels in the whites of the eyes, relaxation and dilation of the bronchial passages, and euphoria.

THC activates the brain's reward system in the same way that other drugs of abuse do, by increasing dopamine levels. Other effects of marijuana include dry mouth, excessive hunger and thirst, sleepiness, and occasionally dysphoria (anxiety, fear, panic, and paranoia). Heavy marijuana use impairs memory and attention. THC also impairs the areas of the brain that regulate balance, posture, coordination of movement, and reaction time.

Intoxication is related to accidents: A significant number of fatal accident victims test positive for THC, either alone or with alcohol. In a study conducted by the National Highway Traffic Safety Administration, it was shown that THC alone impairs driving performance and the effects are even greater when combined with alcohol than for either drug alone.

ECSTASY

A number of illicit drugs commonly used at nightclubs and raves are called "club drugs." Common among these is a drug referred to as Ecstasy (Figure 5.3). Not commonly fatal but

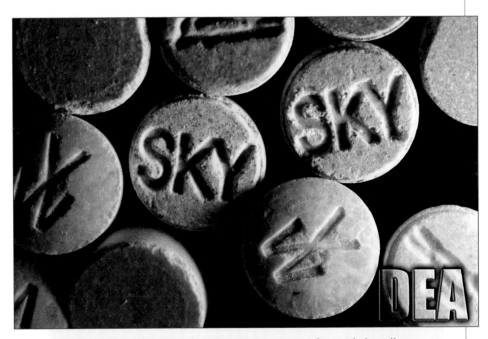

FIGURE 5.3 Ecstasy, the most common name for methylenedioxy-methamphetamine (MDMA), usually comes in a tablet form imprinted with a monogram. A common effect of Ecstasy is an increased feeling of euphoria, and it is notoriously used as a club drug.

important forensically, Ecstasy or MDMA (3,4-methylene-dioxymethamphetamine) is an illegal drug that is classified as both a stimulant and a hallucinogen. MDMA produces stimulant effects similar to those of amphetamines and cocaine, as well as hallucinogenic distortions in time and perception and enhanced tactile (physical or sensory) experiences. It is also known to be an empathy-increasing drug. MDMA is administered orally as a tablet or capsule, and the effects last approximately three to six hours. MDMA is used as a club drug because of its effects as a stimulant, and its sensory and empathy-enhancing properties.

MDMA can affect the brain by altering the activity of certain neurotransmitters, particularly a chemical called serotonin. High doses can be neurotoxic and appear to target serotonin-secreting cells. Damage to these neurons may cause depression, anxiety, memory loss, learning difficulties, sleep disorders, and sexual dysfunction. One of the potentially dangerous side effects of MDMA is hyperthermia (an increase in body temperature), which, on rare occasions, has led to the death of the user. MDMA also causes an increase in heart rate and blood pressure, fainting, panic attacks, and, in severe cases, a loss of consciousness and seizures. It is also known to produce heart arrhythmias, particularly in sensitive individuals, and this has been implicated as a cause in many Ecstasy-related deaths.

Ecstasy tablets also contain other drugs that can be harmful as well. Adulterants found in MDMA include methamphetamine, caffeine, dextromethorphan, ephedrine, and cocaine. Used for its stimulant properties, MDMA is often associated with clubs, dancing, and other vigorous physical activities, usually over prolonged periods. This can potentially lead to a striking rise in body temperature, which can rapidly lead to muscle breakdown and result in kidney failure. Additionally, dehydration, hypertension, and heart failure may occur in predisposed persons.

KETAMINE, PCP, DEXTROMETHORPHAN, AND LSD

Ketamine, PCP (phencyclidine), and dextromethorphan are drugs that have properties known as dissociative anesthetics (Figure 5.4). Ketamine is used as an anesthetic and dextromethorphan is a cough suppressant, while PCP has no current therapeutic use. A dissociative anesthetic is a drug that is used to control pain and anxiety during a surgical procedure but allows the patient to remain conscious. Together with LSD, they can be classified as hallucinogenic drugs. The dissociative drugs act by altering the effects of the neurotransmitter glutamate (perception of pain, responses to the environment, and memory) in the brain.

The only known source of ketamine is via theft and illegal sale of pharmaceutical products from veterinary clinics; some of the drug is diverted from pharmacies in Mexico. Ketamine is injected, smoked, or taken orally in drinks. In its pure form, PCP is a white crystalline powder that is readily dissolved in water or pressed into tablets. PCP usually is sprayed onto tobacco or marijuana cigarettes and smoked. Ketamine and PCP produce similar physical effects and both share some of the visual manifestations of LSD. The drugs produce vivid, colorful hallucinations and what has been described as an out-of-body experience. The drugs can cause delirium, amnesia, depression, and long-term memory and cognitive difficulties. Due to its dissociative effect, ketamine has been reportedly used as a date rape drug. PCP is a particularly dangerous drug because of the wide range of psychological and behavioral effects that it can induce and the unpredictability of the response pattern. PCP is known to affect all of the brain pathways, producing effects ranging from euphoria to anxiety and panic states, and can induce a variety of behavioral patterns. Contrary to popular belief, it does not routinely induce violent behavior, but it is known to release latent aggression in certain individuals.

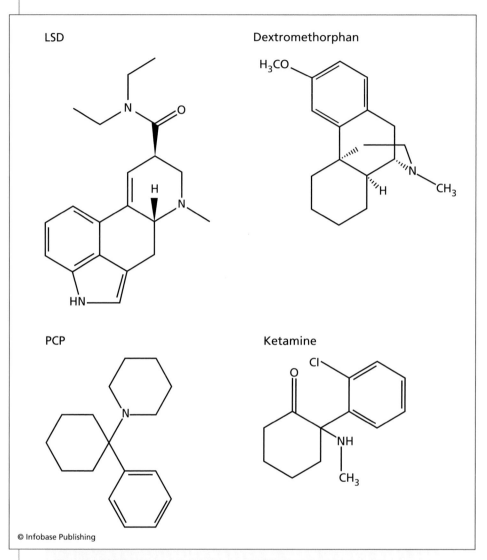

LSD

Dextromethorphan

PCP

Ketamine

FIGURE 5.4 Chemical structures of LSD, PCP, ketamine, and dextromethorphan.

Dextromethorphan is found in over-the-counter cold and cough medications. Like PCP and ketamine, at much higher doses, dextromethorphan acts as a dissociative anesthetic. The effects range from a mild stimulant effect with distorted visual perceptions at low doses to a sense of complete dissociation from one's body at higher doses. These medications also contain antihistamine and decongestant ingredients, which can seriously complicate the risks of dextromethorphan abuse.

LSD (lysergic acid), a Schedule I drug, is a powerful hallucinogenic compound and is primarily manufactured illegally within the United States. Pure LSD is a clear or white, odorless, crystalline material that is water soluble and taken orally. In addition to hallucinations, LSD users may experience panic attacks, mental confusion, paranoia, and anxiety. Flashbacks have been known to occur long after the user has stopped taking the drug. LSD does not produce the same addictive, drug-induced behavior of cocaine and heroin. There are few cases involving fatalities associated with LSD, but it has been implicated in some suicides and accidental deaths during the LSD "trip."

METHAMPHETAMINE

Like cocaine, methamphetamine is a central nervous system stimulant that is highly addictive (Figure 5.5). Methamphetamine is smoked, snorted, injected, or orally ingested. The majority of methamphetamine is produced by Mexican drug traffickers in large clandestine laboratories in Mexico and California. Small laboratories also exist in the Midwest. More recently, there has been increased trafficking of a form of Southeast Asian tablets called "Yaba," containing methamphetamine and caffeine. Methamphetamine use seems to be more common in the West, Southwest, and Midwestern parts of the United States, although it seems to be spreading to the Southeast and Northeast.

Methamphetamine is a white, odorless crystalline solid or powder. The abuse of methamphetamine leads to stimulant

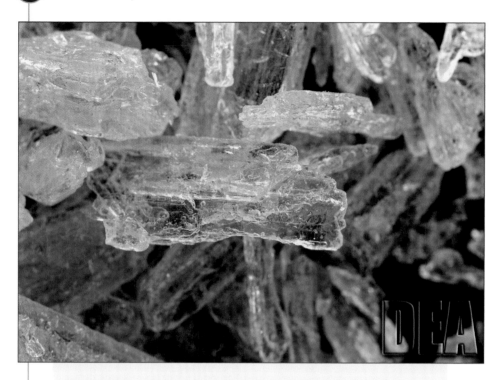

Figure 5.5 Methamphetamine, also known as crystal meth, is a highly addictive psychostimulant drug, which comes in a colorless crystalline form. Short-term effects of meth include heightened mental alertness and loss of fatigue, while long-term use can lead to clinical depression.

effects that are similar to those for cocaine. These effects include aggressive and violent behavior, auditory hallucinations, mood disturbances, delusions, and psychotic and paranoid episodes that can result in homicidal as well as suicidal thoughts. Methamphetamine is neurotoxic in users and dopamine pathways are primarily affected. The potential exists for cardiac and neurological problems, including rapid, irregular heartbeat; hypertension; and stroke. Hyperthermia can also occur with methamphetamine overdoses and, if not treated immediately, can result in death. Due to the secret nature of methamphetamine manufacture, there is always a possibility that it may contain toxic chemical adulterants.

CENTRAL NERVOUS SYSTEM DEPRESSANTS

Central nervous system (CNS) depressants include sedatives, hypnotics (sleep inducing), and antianxiety drugs (tranquilizers). They all slow brain function in a progressive manner and are most often used in the treatment of anxiety and sleep disorders. Among the most common CNS depressants are the following:

- Barbiturates such as secobarbital, phenobarbital, pentobarbital, and amobarbital used to treat seizures, anxiety, tension, and sleep disorders
- **Benzodiazepines** such as diazepam, chlordiazepoxide, lorazepam, triazelam, and alprazolam prescribed to treat anxiety, sleep disorders, and panic attacks

Most CNS depressants act on the brain by facilitating the neurotransmitter gamma-aminobutyric acid (GABA). GABA is an inhibitory neurotransmitter that works by decreasing brain activity. Through their ability to increase GABA activity, CNS depressants produce a sleepy or calming effect.

CNS depressants should not be used in combination with other CNS-depressing drugs. Benzodiazepines are relatively safe medications but can be deadly when combined with alcohol. A CNS depressant alone may cause respiratory depression at high doses, but when two or more are taken together the effects are much greater.

GHB (Gamma-hydroxybutyric Acid)

GHB is a banned Schedule I central nervous system depressant. Originally available in health food stores, it was marketed as a body-building supplement due to its alleged ability to increase production of growth hormones. GHB is easily produced and is still available through illegal channels. Lower doses cause drowsiness, dizziness, nausea, and visual disturbances; at higher dosages, unconsciousness, seizures, severe respiratory depression, coma, and death have been reported.

GHB generates feelings of euphoria and intoxication. It is highly soluble and is primarily available in liquid form. It is often added to flavored beverages to conceal its presence.

Case Study: *Date Rape Drugs*

Aroused by the sound of her front door closing at 5:00 AM, a mother discovered her 15-year-old daughter unconscious on the couch. The girl had been at a party. When her friends were contacted, they said she drank some beer and then wandered off with a man. They had found her about 3:30 AM, in a bedroom, disheveled and acting "zonked." The friends carried her home and deposited her in the living room. The girl was taken to the emergency department where she was groggy but awake. She could remember nothing of the previous evening. Her vital signs were normal, but a pelvic examination suggested recent sexual intercourse. Her blood ethanol level was 22 mg/dL and a urine screen for drugs of abuse was positive only for tetrahydrocannabinol (THC) and ethanol. Later, the result of a test for flunitrazepam (benzodiazepine) returned positive.

Ethanol and pharmaceutical agents are used to sedate potential sexual victims. The use of such agents is a fast-growing problem. Two drugs that have been implicated in

Alcoholic beverages enhance its depressant effects and increase the potential for respiratory depression. GHB has been used as a date rape drug: Slipped into a drink, it causes an unknowing victim to become incapacitated and develops amnesia (memory problems), which complicates any prosecution case. Several victims have died due to this practice, and legislation (the Drug-Induced Rape Prevention and Punishment Act of 1996) to prevent the use of a drug in the commission of a crime has been established.

these crimes are flunitrazepam (Rohypnol®) and gamma-hydroxybutyrate (GHB). Patients under the influence of flunitrazepam will appear intoxicated. Symptoms include slurred speech, impaired judgment, drowsiness, and lethargy. CNS depression to the point of coma may be present particularly if other substances, such as ethanol, have been ingested. The patient will have no memory for the period of intoxication and may still have trouble forming new memory for a while longer.

GHB was originally sold at health food stores for its alleged **anabolic effect**. Now, GHB is manufactured illegally in home labs. GHB is said to make one feel happy, relaxed, and intoxicated. Its memory-erasing effect has led to use as a date rape drug. The onset of symptoms usually occurs within 15 minutes due to rapid gastrointestinal absorption. Small doses may result in relaxation, muscle limpness, and amnesia. Other symptoms include nausea, vomiting, increased urinary frequency, and incontinence. With higher doses, coma and seizure-like symptoms are common.

INHALANTS

Various household and industrial products are used as inhalants due to their psychoactive properties. Inhalants are classified based on their form, such as volatiles, aerosols, gases, and nitrites. Volatile solvents are liquids that vaporize at room temperature and are found in numerous inexpensive, easily available products. The propellants and solvents of aerosol sprays are also abused, as are gases such as medical anesthetics and some household products. Nitrites often are considered a special class of inhalants and are used primarily as sexual enhancers. Nitrites act primarily to dilate blood vessels and relax the muscles.

Inhalants are often the first drugs that young children experiment with. About 3% of U.S. children have tried inhalants by the time they reach the fourth grade and inhalant abuse can

Table 5.3 Inhalant Classification

INHALANT	EXAMPLES
Volatiles	Paint thinner, felt-tip markers, liquid paper, gasoline, glues, dry-cleaning fluid, degreasers
Gases	Ether, chloroform, halothane, nitrous oxide, butane, propane, refrigerants
Aerosols	Spray paints, deodorant sprays, hair spray, vegetable oil sprays for cooking, and fabric protector sprays
Nitrites	Amyl nitrite, isobutyl nitrite, cyclohexl nitrite, video head cleaner, leather cleaner, liquid aroma

become chronic and extend into adulthood. Inhalants can be breathed in through the nose or the mouth in a variety of ways. Inhaled chemicals are rapidly absorbed through the lungs and delivered to the brain via the bloodstream. Shortly after inhaling the substance, the person experiences intoxicating CNS-depressing effects similar to those produced by alcohol. These include euphoria, intoxication with initial excitation, disinhibition, motor function impairment, impaired judgment, slurred speech, dizziness, nausea and vomiting, hallucinations, and delusions. Coma and death are possible with heavy use.

One of the most common active agents found in inhalants is toluene, which has been shown to activate the brain's dopamine system. Therefore, inhalants containing toluene could become habit forming due to dopamine's role in rewarding behavior. Inhalants are neurotoxic and brain damage is known to occur with their use; permanent injury is a likely outcome with prolonged exposure. Also, a syndrome known as sudden sniffing death may occur, probably due to cardiac arrhythmias that may develop following a single use. Sudden sniffing death is most often associated with the use of butane, propane, and aerosols. Additionally, inhalant abuse can cause fatal asphyxiation, suffocation, convulsions and seizures, choking, and accidents from driving while impaired.

Postmortem Forensic Toxicology

The only thing necessary for the triumph of evil is for good men to do nothing.

—Edmund Burke (1729–1797)

Any violent, unnatural, sudden, or unexpected death is investi-gated by the **medical examiner** or coroner's office to establish the cause and manner of death. The cause of death is the disease, injury, or intoxication that resulted in the person dying. The manner of death is classified as homicide, suicide, accidental, or natural. The investigation includes all the information surrounding the case history and the results from an autopsy (pathological, histological, and toxicological findings). The role of the forensic toxicologist is to provide the necessary information to answer the question: "Did drugs or poisons play a role in the person's death?" In general, a case falls under the jurisdiction of a medical examiner's office when the death:

- Resulted from violent, criminal, suicidal, or accidental means, including any death from criminal neglect or due to suspicious or unexplained activity.

- Occurs in an apparently healthy person with no explained causes.
- Occurs during certain medical procedures.
- Is a fetal or still birth.
- Occurs with no attending physician present.
- Occurs when a person is incarcerated or confined.
- May have been caused by drugs or chemical poisoning.

Therefore, any unnatural death that cannot be explained by a medically recognized disease may be referred to the medical examiner for investigation.

LOOKING FOR CLUES

The forensic pathologist has the primary responsibility for determining the manner and cause of death of a person. In suspected drug and poisoning deaths, the pathologist collects and preserves the specimens for toxicological analysis subsequent to the autopsy. This is the first step in what is known as the chain of custody. Maintaining the integrity of the samples is vital to achieve reliability and confidence in the results. Forensic work is held to a legal standard, so it is under close scrutiny regarding the handling of the toxicology specimens.

Sometimes there are clues or telltale signs that point to a specific poison, such as curious smells (e.g., cyanide) or certain characteristic pathological findings. Some cases are submitted to toxicology with no clues as to what the offending agent could be and the approach is that of a general unknown. The case history and investigation may help to narrow the search, but this is not always possible. Testing must rule out as many substances as possible, because negative results often are just as important to the case as positive ones. For example, the lack of a life-sustaining drug may play a role in a death just as easily as the presence of a toxic drug.

Most toxicology laboratories have established protocols for dealing with different types of cases. The following are examples of possible toxicological scenarios dealt with daily in forensic medicine:

- Drug overdose

- Homicide by poison

- The role of alcohol impairment in an accident or crime

- If drugs such as antidepressants were used in suicide

- Determining if assertions of self-defense against drug-induced psychotic behavior are plausible

- If drugs were used to incapacitate a victim of a crime

- Whether a patient was in compliance with their prescribed medicines

- Some other, yet unknown cause of death

SAMPLE PREPARATION

Specimen selection, collection, and preservation play an enormously important role in toxicology. The old saying "garbage in, garbage out" applies to toxicology better than to any other science. Attempting to perform accurate analyses in the laboratory with improper specimens is like trying to make a cake with the wrong ingredients. The expectation is for the forensic laboratory to produce quality and legally defensible results, and this depends upon the proper collection and storage of specimens.

The challenge with postmortem samples is that the quality and availability of the samples themselves can vary greatly. Unlike testing clinical samples from living individuals, postmortem toxicology has the unique problem of testing samples collected at autopsy that may have undergone varying levels of decomposition. There are several approaches to improving or maintaining the quality of autopsy samples. The use of proper preservatives is important to prevent further postmortem changes in the samples. Even the selection of the container itself can be important. For example, some drugs will adhere to glass causing erroneously low results. Glass containers may require specialized treatment prior to their use to prevent this from happening. In addition, care must be taken because glass containers can break and the sample may be lost. Plastic containers have their problems as well: Some plastics may release contaminating chemicals into the specimens and alter the results. Also, how the container is sealed is important because volatile agents can be lost if the seal is not airtight. It is a tricky set of problems that has required testing and research to come up with the best solutions.

Another important consideration is that some agents are not stable in postmortem samples and may be lost over time. Conversely, some drug or poison levels can actually increase in postmortem specimens if allowed to stand without proper care. They may be temperature sensitive and require cold storage or they be susceptible to the action of microorganisms present in the samples. Preservatives like sodium fluoride for blood are used to inhibit the effects of microorganisms and all samples are refrigerated to retard the growth of bacteria and prevent the loss of volatile drugs and poisons. Clearly, what seems like a simple task becomes much more complicated when all factors are considered.

The proper specimen must be used to assemble all the pieces of the puzzle when trying to determine a cause and manner of death. For example, urine may be an excellent sample to screen for the presence of drugs or metabolites. It is easy to work with, and it is the major pathway for the excretion of most drugs and

Table 6.1 Postmortem Samples Collected for Toxicology

SAMPLE	CONSIDERATIONS
Blood	Specimen of choice for interpretation of toxicological findings. In general, peripheral blood should be used because for many drugs there is postmortem redistribution to heart blood, which is not reflective of levels prior to death. Drugs may concentrate in plasma or the red blood cells.
Urine	Good for qualitative information on past exposure or use. Specimen most often used for screening, but not used for assessment of impairment or intoxication. High concentration of drug metabolites.
Bile	Also useful for qualitative screening. Drugs may be found at higher concentrations than in blood. Most often used for detecting opiates and morphine.
Vitreous Humor	Less subject to contamination and not affected by embalming. Not used in cases of decomposition. Used to estimate antemortem alcohol in embalmed bodies and to assess other important antemortem physiological functions.
Gastric Contents	Following oral administration, may find undissolved capsules or tablets in stomach contents. A large quantity of drug in the stomach is indicative of oral overdose. Odors may be present that give a clue of agents present.
Tissues	Liver, kidney, brain, lung, and spleen are commonly collected at autopsy. Used along with blood to interpret findings. Some poisons such as metals will accumulate in tissues. Lung is useful for volatile substances, brain for fat-soluble agents, and spleen for compounds with affinity for red blood cells.
Hair	Used for historical and past exposure. Long window of detection, but may be subject to external contamination.

Table 6.1 Postmortem Samples Collected for Toxicology	
SAMPLE	CONSIDERATIONS
Bone	Some metals accumulate in bone; marrow may provide a sample when other specimens are unavailable due to decomposition. Drugs have been identified in skeletonized remains.
Skeletal Muscle	Available and well preserved for longer period of time after death and may provide information in decomposed cases.
Other Samples	Fly larvae (maggots), blood stains, soil samples, and cremation ash are among other samples that may contain drugs or poisons. Tablets, capsules, vials, and various household products may be collected at the scene.

poisons and therefore can have easily detectable quantities of the agent. However, its use in interpretation of intoxication or impairment is not possible because many drugs or their metabolites may be present in the urine for hours, days, or even weeks after use. Furthermore, a drug may be present in urine without being present in blood. Blood is the better sample choice for determining impairment. Accordingly, urine is often used to screen for the presence of a drug and confirmation and quantification are done in the blood and/or other tissues.

LABORATORY ANALYSIS

Once the samples have been collected and properly preserved, the next step involves the separation of the analytes (the substances you want to measure) from the biological matter. This is referred to as the extraction procedure. Most specimens require a certain degree of pretreatment and isolation of the drug or poison. The exception to this generality is urine, which can usually be used for the direct analysis of drugs without exhaustive preparation. In order to isolate the drug or poison, proteins and other interfering components must be removed from the sample prior to analysis. This is accomplished by a variety of methods. Distillation, protein precipitation, liquid-liquid extraction, and solid-phase extraction (SPE) are some of the common methods used in toxicology.

The methods of analysis include spectrophotometry, chromatography, and immunoassay techniques, along with confirmatory procedures of which mass spectrometry is the most common.

Spectrophotometry

The simplest example of spectrophotometric analysis would be a simple color test. Color tests allow for rapid presumptive identification of a drug or poison based on a color change in the sample solution following the addition of a reagent. Salicylate, cyanide, and acetaminophen are substances that can be screened by use of a color test. Ultraviolet spectrophotometry is an instrumental spectrophotometric screening method that has also been used in forensic toxicology laboratories. It was very a popular method that was included in most toxicology protocols for several decades. While this method is still available to the toxicologist, it has largely been replaced by other more sensitive and specific tests.

Chromatography

Chromatography is one of the primary methods used in forensic toxicology. There are several types of chromatography, including thin-layer chromatography, gas chromatography (GC), and liquid chromatography (LC). GC and LC are very popular in forensic toxicology because they are easy to use, sensitive, and

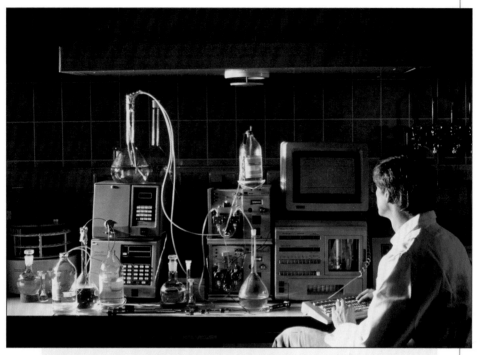

FIGURE 6.1 In this photograph, a chemist is using high performance liquid chromatography (HPLC) equipment in order to separate mixtures of molecules. This method is particularly good at separating large biological molecules, such as proteins, as well as many drugs.

provide good initial separations. The advantage of these methods is that several instrumental parameters can be modified to enhance their performance based upon the chemical nature of the drugs or substances to be analyzed.

Chromatography allows for the separation of individual compounds present in a sample extract. This is based on dissolving the sample in a mobile phase, usually a gas (GC) or liquid (LC), and then passing it through an immobile (stationary) phase. The phases are selected to produce different solubilities in the sample components, separating them from one another depending on how slowly or quickly they pass through. If a component is more soluble in the stationary phase, it will take longer for it to pass through. Conversely, if it is more soluble in the mobile phase it will pass through much faster. Methods such as gas chromatography and high performance liquid chromatography (HPLC) employ this principle. GC and HPLC use columns which are packed with the stationary phase and the mobile phase (Figure 6.1). As the mobile phase exits the column the separated components will elute at different times based upon the speed at which the substance moves through the system. This time is referred to as the retention time. Different substances have different retention times and these can be compared to those of a known standard compound. Quantification can also be accomplished by comparing the response (peaks) of the unknown agent to that of known quantities of the standards.

The gold standard of confirmatory techniques is gas chromatography/mass spectrometry (GC/MS) or liquid chromatography/mass spectrometry (LC/MS). A sample's spectrum can be compared to an extensive library of mass spectra for known compounds to provide a suitable match. Quantification of the drug or poison is done by GC, LC, or MS. The end result of the analytic process is useful data on the identity and concentrations of a drug or poison in postmortem samples. Based on this information, the toxicologist can answer questions about the role of a drug or poison in establishing a cause of death.

IMMUNOASSAY

Immunoassays are also popular techniques used for screening in forensic toxicology (Figure 6.2). Immunoassay is a tool for determining the presumptive presence of a drug or class of drugs in biological samples. Immunoassays use antibodies that bind with a target compound or class of compounds, in this case, drugs. This technology has been used widely for screening in

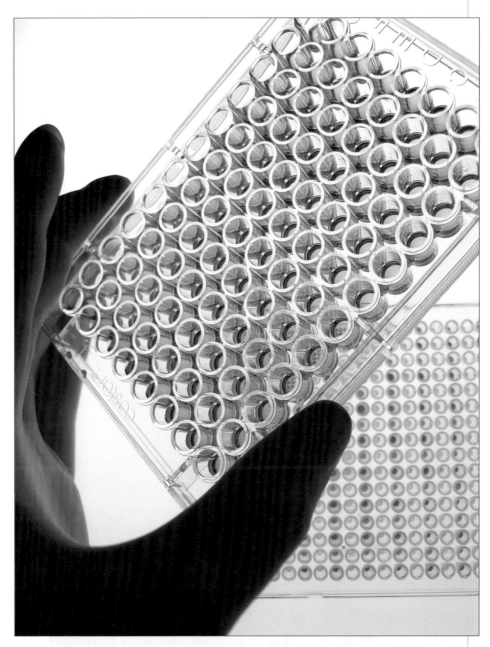

FIGURE 6.2 Pictured above is a sample tray during an enzyme-linked immunosorbent assay (ELISA) blood test. This test is used to detect an antibody or antigen in a blood sample.

toxicology because the methods are relatively fast and straight-forward to use. Concentrations of analytes are identified, for example, by comparing the color of the unknown drug concentration with the color of a standard drug concentration, using a spectrophotometer.

Immunoassays are often performed directly on urine specimens, while others may require protein-free samples that have undergone separation and preparation. They are directed toward detection of a specific drug or class of drugs.

These are types of immunoassay:

- Enzyme-multiplied immunoassay (EMIT)
- Radioimmunoassay (RIA)
- Fluorescent polarization immunoassay (FPIA)
- Kinetic interaction of microparticles in solution immunoassay (KIMS)
- Enzyme-linked immunosorbent assay (ELISA)

EMIT and ELISA are probably used most often for toxicological analysis, because of their speed, sensitivity, selectivity, and lack of radioactive materials. Immunoassays are easy to use, relatively low cost per sample, and cover a range of drugs or drug classes. However, care must be taken if similar compounds to the target are present, as interference and cross-reactivity may generate false positive results. Therefore, all presumptively positive immunoassay results must be confirmed by mass spectrometry.

Drug Testing

Good people do not need laws to tell them to act responsibly, while bad people will find a way around the laws.
                                    —Plato (428–347 B.C.)

During the last two decades, workplace drug testing has become common and approximately 30 million Americans are tested each year for illegal drug use. Recreational drug use continues to be a significant problem and forensic drug screening is a viable method for determining the extent of drug abuse in individuals in the workforce and in schools. Drug testing is used by the military, criminal justice system, and the public and private sectors as a way to monitor health status and to protect the public from the harmful consequences of drug use in certain vital jobs. The U.S. military, transportation workers and pilots, a large percentage of Fortune 500 companies' workforces, various criminal justice agencies, and segments of the manufacturing and utility workers industry regularly screen their applicants for drug use.

Individuals undergo preemployment testing, random or periodic testing, and testing as part of accident investigations. Employers may test potential job applicants to identify individuals that may pose a safety risk, or they may establish random drug testing of employees to detect current drug use, or as a deterrent to drug use, among the staff. As part of accident investigations, drug screening is often used to exclude drug abuse as a contributing factor. Forensic drug testing is also employed by the criminal justice system and law enforcement agencies to determine the role of drugs in various criminal activities.

The first to establish drug testing programs was the U.S. military. In the early 1970s, testing was started because of the fear that drug use could impact the preparedness of its combat forces. Testing procedures were developed to detect drug use and to provide a drug-free workplace in the military. Recruits must undergo drug screening prior to and during their entire military careers.

Drug testing is also used to monitor drug use in the criminal justice and prison system. Criminal offenders are tested regularly to determine their involvement with drugs. Some are tested at arrest and others are also tested while in prison. Most criminal justice systems also require drug testing for persons on probation and as a condition of parole.

Drug testing also has been extended to the sports community. It seems you cannot turn on the television or radio without hearing something about a professional athlete using performance-enhancing drugs, from baseball players using anabolic steroids to runners using blood-**doping** agents (Figure 7.1). Even doping of racehorses has become a problem and equine drug-testing programs have been developed as a result. Both professional and Olympic drug-testing protocols have been established to determine the extent of drug use, but the real concern over performance-enhancing drugs is their increasing popularity in high school athletes. Testing programs are currently being developed to include these agents as a matter of ensuring the health of these younger athletes.

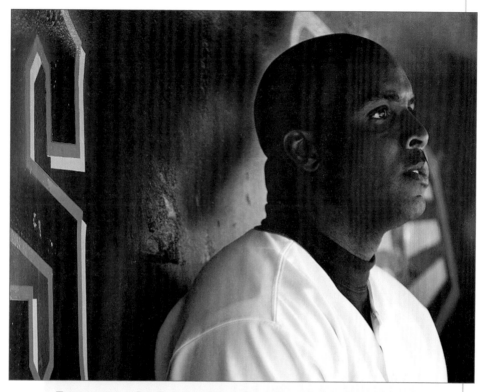

FIGURE 7.1 San Francisco Giants' star Barry Bonds sits in the dugout during a game against the San Diego Padres in June 2001. Bonds, who holds many MLB records including most home runs in a single season, has been accused of taking steroids, although he has never failed a drug test.

REGULATION OF DRUG TESTING

With the rapid growth of drug testing, it became apparent that some form of regulation was needed. Regulated testing in the public and private sectors began in 1983 when the National Transportation Safety Board, the Federal Railway Administration, and the National Institute on Drug Abuse (**NIDA**) developed regulations for the U.S. Department of Transportation. Many companies, particularly those involved in the transportation industry and others that had employees in sensitive positions, began to establish their own drug testing programs. Eventually, the federal government became involved and, in 1986, the National Institute on Drug Abuse (NIDA) convened a conference. Consensus was reached regarding the circumstances under which testing could be conducted. The following points were agreed to:

- All individuals must be informed that they are to be tested.
- The results must be confidential.
- All positive results must be confirmed by an alternate method.
- Properly administered random drug screening is appropriate and legally defensible.

The NIDA conference provided the early foundation upon which much of the technical, legal, and ethical issues developed into the programs that exist today. Drug testing has continued to evolve, and reliable testing is now expected and required. Strict standards must be adhered to and regular assessment of the test laboratories' performance is routinely carried out. Forensic drug testing has become a major force in curbing recreational drug use in many populations.

TESTING PRINCIPLES AND STRATEGIES

As with postmortem testing, forensic drug screening must be approached with the idea that the results may be subject to litigation. The quality of the results will surely be scrutinized, as they can be the difference between a person being hired or fired. Drug testing also has a legal basis because the results can be part of an investigation of an accident or a criminal activity.

Forensic drug testing begins with collection of the sample and ends with the generation of a report. Collection sites and laboratories must follow rigorous forensic toxicology standards regarding collection procedures, specimen integrity, transportation, and the proper safeguarding. Traditionally, the vast majority of forensic testing protocols call for the use of urine as the specimen used for screening. Urine is used because it provides information on past use of drugs and many drugs and their metabolites can be detected in urine in significant quantities for prolonged periods. However, the Substance Abuse and Mental Health Services Administration (SAMHSA) has proposed a new rule that would allow federal agencies to use sweat, saliva, and hair in drug testing programs that now test only urine. For human performance toxicology and assessment of

Table 7.1 Detection Periods for Drugs or Metabolites in Urine

SUBSTANCE	DETECTION TIME
Alcohol	24 hours
Amphetamines	2 to 3 days
Barbiturates (except phenobarbital)	2 to 3 days
Phenobarbital	7 to 14 days
Cannabis (single use)	1 to 3 days
Cannabis (habitual use)	Up to 84 days
Cocaine	1 to 3 days
Heroin	2 to 3 days
LSD	2 to 24 hours

Drummer, O.H. *Forensic Aspects of Drugs of Abuse*. New York: Oxford University Press, 2001.

impairment, blood is collected and used for the analysis. Blood must be used since urine cannot be used to determine timing of drug consumption or to estimate the level of intoxication.

Most commonly, forensic drug testing requires that the individual provide a urine (or blood, hair, or saliva) sample to an employer, medical professional, or law enforcement agent. The sample is properly sealed and sent to a laboratory for testing. Sometimes, the drug test is completed on-site (workplace, school, or at home), often using a commercially available rapid test kit. These types of tests provide presumptive information and must be confirmed by an accredited laboratory if they are to be defensible in court.

THE NIDA FIVE

The so-called NIDA five are five major drugs of abuse that are commonly screened in drug testing laboratories in the United States. The drug testing guidelines that were formerly under the direction of the National Institute on Drug Abuse (NIDA) are currently regulated by the Substance Abuse and Mental Health Services Administration (SAMHSA). SAMHSA requires that certain transportation personnel and those in sensitive occupations are tested for the presence of five specific drug groups:

- Cannabinoids (marijuana, hashish)
- Cocaine (cocaine, crack, benzoylecognine)
- Amphetamines (amphetamines, methamphetamine, speed)
- Opiates (heroin, opium, codeine, morphine)
- Phencyclidine (PCP)

Most toxicology laboratories test for a much wider range of drugs and will add additional drugs to the screen upon request.

Benzodiazepines, barbiturates, MDMA, GHB, fentanyl, ketamine, LSD, and others may be part of a more comprehensive drug screen. They may not be included as part of a preemployment test because of added expense and employers generally just screen for the NIDA five.

TESTING PROCEDURE

Upon arrival at the laboratory the sample's integrity is checked and it is processed for analysis. Urine is screened by using appropriate methods for the presence of the drugs. A two-step process is used that includes a screening test followed by a confirmation test using an alternative method for any positive results. The most common screening methods employed are immunoassays. These allow for the sensitive detection of specific drugs or drug classes in a rapid, easy, and efficient manner. No extraction is needed and minimum sample preparation is required. These tests are available in commercial kits. Some of the drawbacks of immunoassay are that they may be susceptible to adulteration, which can result in a false negative, or they are subject to possible false positives because of cross-reacting substances in the specimen. Because these tests can be prone to false positive results, confirmation is required. The confirmation test that most labs use is gas chromatography/mass spectrometry. Known drug standards and controls are analyzed along with the specimens to check the accuracy and precision of the methods used.

In addition to urine testing, drug testing on hair is becoming more popular due to its long window of detection. Based upon a number of factors including growth rates, drugs can be detected in the hair for six months or longer. Most laboratories use segments of hair within 3–5 centimeters (1.2 to 2 inches) of the scalp, which limits the detection window to about 90 days.

Saliva drug tests can generally detect drug use during the previous few days and have several advantages. They are a non-invasive method, the sample cannot be adulterated, and saliva tests are particularly suited for on-site testing. Saliva-

The Limits of Drug Tests

When seeking to identify drugs of abuse in patients, physicians should know the limits of drug tests that they perform. Most urine screens for drugs of abuse test for opiates, tetrahydro-cannabinol (marijuana), benzoylecgonine (cocaine), amphetamines, and sometimes phencyclidine. Other drugs of abuse, including GHB, LSD, the alkaloids in Jimson weed, and the toxins in psilocybin mushrooms, will not be detected unless they are specifically looked for. Unfortunately, even some drugs within the classes screened do not show up. These include flunitrazepam, a benzodiazepine; MDMA, an amphetamine derivative; and several opiates: methadone, oxycodone, pentazocine, and fentanyl derivatives. Sedative hypnotics of other classes, including zolpidem and chloral hydrate, and centrally acting muscle relaxants such as cyclobenzaprine (Flexeril®) will not be detected. Comprehensive drug screening will detect methadone, zolpidem, cyclobenzaprine, and pentazocine but not some of the other substances previously mentioned. Specific drug testing can identify flunitrazepam, chloral hydrate, LSD, MDMA, GHB, and oxycodone but only if the physician names the suspected agent and specifically requests that gas chromatography with mass spectrometry (GC/MS) be performed. No tests are available for psilocybin mushroom or Jimson weed toxins.

based tests are as accurate as urine screens and in many cases closely mimic results found with blood; they can be implemented to determine intoxication. Research regarding the use of saliva to infer the degree of impairment is currently controversial.

Sweat patches designed to detect drugs collected in sweat over a two-week period are sometimes employed when there is a desire to monitor drug use over a prolonged time course (e.g., in parolees). The patches are removed after the test period and analyzed for the presence of drugs.

HUMAN PERFORMANCE TOXICOLOGY

Human performance toxicology is the assessment of the ability to perform routine psychomotor tasks in the face of impairing agents, such as alcohol or drugs. These factors determine the ability of a person to perform such tasks as driving a car or performing on the job and have important legal implications. It involves the effective use of the brain functions to control coordination and motor skills required on the highway and in the workplace. Forensic toxicologists have become interested in performance-based toxicology due to the legal implications of drug use. Human performance may be enhanced, which is the basis of performance-enhancing drugs in sports, or degraded, such as driving under the influence of drugs or alcohol.

Whether it is alcohol, heroin, GHB, antidepressants, or benzodiazepines, drug use can alter one's ability to perform tasks required to safely operate a vehicle, fly a plane, pilot a ship, or walk on a steel beam 20 stories up, and so on. Based on the pharmacological effects of a drug, product warnings may be issued on the risk involved in driving a car or operating machinery while under the influence of drugs. For illicit drugs, warnings either do not exist or are of no consequence. There are established procedures for determining the effect of drugs on human performance, including standardized field sobriety tests, drug recognition experts (DRE) evaluation and field testing (e.g., alcohol breath testing), and laboratory analysis.

SPORTS TESTING

The use of drugs and medications by athletes has been a problem for a long time. Performance-enhancing drugs are designed to provide an advantage in athletics. The practice is referred to as doping and affects the body in different ways, such as increasing muscle mass, strength, or the capacity of the blood to carry oxygen. Doping will give a competitive advantage to the athlete, but at the cost of some very dangerous consequences.

The use of doping agents is as old as competitive sports itself. Stories date back to the ancient Olympics in Greece of athletes attempting to use methods to enhance athletic performance. This practice still lives on today. However, due to possible health problems and ethical reasons, the International Olympic Committee agreed to ban and/or restrict performance-enhancing substances in 1967 and methods to detect their use have since been developed.

Doping substances are generally banned because of:

- Health reasons: Many performance-enhancing drugs can have serious, even fatal, effects. Many of these drugs have been banned due to their high potential to cause toxicity and other negative consequences on human health.

- Ethical reasons: The idea that performance-enhancing drugs offer an advantage above the basic ability of the athlete's natural levels is considered cheating.

- Legal reasons: Many agents on the banned list are illegal drugs. They may serve the role of enhancing performance (e.g., narcotics for pain) or the athlete may simply abuse them.

Some reasons a person uses performance-enhancing drugs are obvious, including dissatisfaction with athletic performance or progress, low self-esteem, inflated ego, pressure to win (from coaches, parents, media, and the public), monetary rewards, and high performance expectations. It is most often a combination of factors that leads an athlete to doping. However, one of the frightening trends is the increased misuse of drugs by younger athletes to gain a competitive edge in sports or simply because they want to look better.

Even with the knowledge that these substances are harmful, the use of performance-enhancing drugs and the demand for such substances has skyrocketed. The height of the problem has become evident with the current evidence that use in teenage athletes is escalating. In fact, not only athletes but also others outside of sports are now seeking performance-enhancing drugs to improve their physical appearance. Currently, there are estimates that more than one million high school students have used steroids, and the numbers are growing.

An important forensic aspect of steroid abuse is the reported increase in aggressive behavior with steroids. Increased acts of violence, suicide, robbery, and other dangerous acts have been attributed to steroid abuse. In addition, various cardiovascular, liver, and skin disorders have also been reported with steroid use.

The World Anti-Doping Agency (WADA)

One of the most important agencies that is involved in the adoption of anti-doping rules is the World Anti-Doping Agency. They developed the code that is the core document

Table 7.2 Banned Drugs in Sports

CLASS	PURPOSE	METHOD OF TESTING
Stimulants	To increase alertness and reduce fatigue during competition	GC, GC/MS
Narcotics	To reduce pain during training and competition	GC, GC/MS
Anabolic Agents/ Steroids	To increase muscle strength and bulk during training	GC, GC/MS
Diuretics	To lose weight quickly; to evade doping tests by diluting urine	GC, GC/MS
Peptide hormones and related substances	To increase muscle strength and bulk; to increase endurance	LC/MS and immunoassays

for anti-doping policies, rules, and regulations within sports organizations and among public authorities. WADA has identified a list of classes of agents that are banned by participating sports organizations. These include stimulants, narcotics,

EXAMPLES	HEALTH CONSIDERATIONS
Amphetamines, caffeine, cocaine, ephedrine	Increased heart rate and can impact the body's ability to regulate temperature
Heroin, morphine, methadone, opium	CNS depression, addiction, respiratory depression
Androgenic anabolic steroids (artificial versions of the male hormone testosterone), testosterone, nandrolone, beta-2 agonists (nonsteroidal)	Users risk liver damage, baldness, acne, excessive hair growth on the face and back, changes in sexual characteristics (males exhibiting some female characteristics and vice versa), and potential infertility.
Dexatrim, mannitol	Increased urine production can make an athlete susceptible to dehydration.
Human growth hormone (HGH), erythropoietin (EPO)	Growth hormones: acromegaly (athlete's hands, feet, and face grow very large), problems with joints and muscles, diabetes Erythropoietin (taken to stimulate red blood cell production for endurance purposes): an increase in blood viscosity, potential for cardiovascular problems

anabolic agents/steroids, diuretics, peptide hormones and related compounds, and other restricted drugs. Each of these classes includes hundreds of compounds. Most international sports associations and professional sports leagues abide by the WADA guidelines (see Table 7.2)

The most commonly tested biological sample is urine, for the reasons discussed earlier. Some types of drugs are difficult to detect in urine, so blood samples are preferred. Athletes can be tested randomly or in connection with a specific athletic competition (e.g., the Olympics). Three testing methodologies make up the bulk of the drug testing: gas chromatography (GC), liquid chromatography (LC), and mass spectrometry (MS).

GLOSSARY

Addiction   A chronic, relapsing disease characterized by compulsive drug seeking and use, despite harmful consequences, and by neurochemical and molecular changes in the brain.

Anabolic steroids   Synthetic substances related to the male sex hormones (androgens). They promote the growth of skeletal muscle (anabolic effects) and the development of male sexual characteristics (androgenic effects).

Analgesics   A group of medications that reduce pain.

Anoxia   Absence of oxygen; a pathological deficiency of oxygen.

Autopsy   Examination of a cadaver to determine or confirm the cause of death; also called necropsy, postmortem, and postmortem examination.

Barbiturate   A type of CNS depressant often prescribed to promote sleep.

Benzodiazepine   A type of CNS depressant often prescribed to relieve anxiety. Valium and Librium are among the most widely prescribed medications.

Cannabinoids   Chemicals that help control mental and physical processes when produced naturally by the body and that produce intoxication and other effects when absorbed from marijuana.

Carboxyhemoglobin   The compound that is formed when inhaled carbon monoxide combines with hemoglobin, binding more tightly than oxygen and rendering the hemoglobin incapable of transporting oxygen.

Central nervous system (CNS)   The brain and spinal cord.

CNS depressants   A class of drugs that slow CNS function (also called sedatives and tranquilizers), some of which are used to treat anxiety and sleep disorders; includes barbiturates and benzodiazepines.

Cocaethylene   Potent stimulant created when cocaine and alcohol are used together.

Confirmational analysis   Analytical method used to confirm the presence of drugs or chemicals in specimens following a positive screening test.

Dopamine   A neurotransmitter present in regions of the brain that regulate movement, emotion, motivation, and feelings of pleasure.

Doping   The use by athletes of banned substances or methods that may enhance performance.

Glossary

Embalmed   Treated (a corpse) with preservatives in order to prevent decay.

Euphoria   An exaggerated feeling of physical and mental well-being, especially when not justified by external reality. It may be induced by drugs such as opioids, amphetamines, and alcohol and is also a feature of mania.

Extraction   The process of obtaining or isolating something from a mixture, compound, or tissue by chemical or physical or mechanical means.

Forensic toxicology   Discipline encompassing the measurement of alcohol, drugs, and other toxic substances in biological specimens and interpretation of such results in a medicolegal context.

General unknown   A case in which there is no known cause of death and no history that indicates what drug or toxin may be present in a deceased individual.

Homicidal poisoning   The killing of one person by another by the use of chemical means.

Hormone   A chemical substance formed in glands in the body and carried in the blood to organs and tissues, where it influences function, structure, and behavior.

Hyoscine   A drug also known as scopolamine. It is obtained from the nightshade plant.

Medical examiner   A physician officially authorized by a governmental unit to ascertain the cause of death, especially those not occurring under natural circumstances.

Metabolites   A substance produced by metabolism.

NIDA   National Institute on Drug Abuse.

Opioid   Controlled drugs or narcotics most often prescribed for the management of pain; natural or synthetic chemicals based on opium's active component, morphine, that work by mimicking the actions of pain-relieving chemicals produced in the body.

Physical dependence   An adaptive physiological state that can occur with regular drug use and results in withdrawal when drug use is discontinued. (Physical dependence alone is not the same as addiction, which involves compulsive drug seeking and use, despite its harmful consequences.)

Poison   Any agent capable of producing harm in a biological system.

Postmortem redistribution   The diffusion (movement) of a drug or poison from its location in the body at the time of death to another location during the postmortem period (interval between time of death and autopsy).

Preliminary screening tests   Presumptive and rapid qualitative methods to detect the presence of drugs.

Psychoactive   Having a specific effect on the mind.

Qualitative analysis   Determination of what drug or poison was present.

Quantitative analysis   Measurement of the level of poison present.

Respiratory depression   Suppression of breathing that results in the reduced availability of oxygen to vital organs.

Sedatives   Drugs that suppress anxiety and relax muscles, including benzodiazepines, barbiturates, and other types of CNS depressants.

Stimulant   Drug that increases or enhances the activity of monoamines (such as dopamine and norepinephrine) in the brain, which leads to increased heart rate, blood pressure, and respiration; used to treat only a few disorders, such as narcolepsy and attention deficit.

THC (Delta-9-tetrahydrocannabinol)   The main active ingredient in marijuana, which acts on the brain to produce its effects.

Tolerance   A condition in which higher doses of a drug are required to produce the same effects as experienced initially.

Toxic   Temporary or permanent drug effects that are detrimental to the functioning of an organ or group of organs.

Tranquilizers   Drugs prescribed to promote sleep or reduce anxiety, including benzodiazepines, barbiturates, and other types of CNS depressants.

Withdrawal   A variety of symptoms that occur after chronic use of some drug is reduced or stopped.

BIBLIOGRAPHY

Abraham, H.D., A.M. Aldridge, and P. Gogia. "The Psychopharmacology of Hallucinogens." *Neuropsychopharmacology* 14 (1996): 285–298.

Aghajanian, G.K., and G.J. Marek. "Serotonin and Hallucinogens." *Neuropsychopharmacology* 21 (1999): 16S–23S.

Bahrke, M.S., C.E. Yesalis, and J.E. Wright. "Psychological and Behavioral Effects of Endogenous Testosterone and Anabolic-androgenic Steroids: An Update." *Sports Medicine* 22:6 (1996): 367–390.

Balster, R.L. "Neural Basis of Inhalant Abuse." *Drug and Alcohol Dependence* 51:1–2 (1998): 207–214.

Bartrip, P. "A 'Pennurth of Arsenic for Rat Poison': The Arsenic Act, 1851 and the Prevention of Secret Poisoning." *Medical History* 36:1 (1992): 53–69.

Block, R.I., and M.M. Ghoneim. "Effects of Chronic Marijuana Use on Human Cognition." *Psychopharmacology* 100:1–2 (1993): 219–228.

"Blood Alcohol Estimator." Distributed by The Traffic Institute, Northwest University, 1986.

Blue, J.G., and J.A. Lombardo. "Steroids and Steroid-like Compounds." *Clinics in Sports Medicine* 18:3 (1999): 667–689.

Bolla, K.I., U.D. McCann, and G.A. Ricaurte. "Memory Impairment in Abstinent MDMA ('Ecstasy') Users." *Neurology* 51 (1998): 1532–1537.

Bronson, F.H., and C.M. Matherne. "Exposure to Anabolic-androgenic Steroids Shortens Life Span of Male Mice." *Medicine and Science in Sports and Exercise* 29:5 (1997): 615–619.

Brower, K.J. "Withdrawal from Anabolic Steroids." *Current Therapy in Endocrinology and Metabolism* 6 (1997): 338–343.

Christophersen, A.S. "Amphetamine Designer Drugs: An Overview and Epidemiology." *Toxicology Letters* 112–113 (2000): 127–131.

Cimbura, G., D.M. Lucas, R.C. Bennett, and A.C. Donelson. "Incidence and Toxicological Aspects of Cannabis and Ethanol Detected in 1,394 Fatally Injured Drivers and Pedestrians in Ontario (1982–1984)." *Journal of Forensic Science* 35:5 (1990): 1035–1041.

Colado, M.I., E. O'Shea, R. Granados, et al. "A Study of the Neurotoxic Effect of MDMA ('Ecstasy') on 5-HT Neurons in the Brains of Mothers and

Neonates Following Administration of the Drug During Pregnancy." *British Journal of Pharmacology* 121 (1997): 827–833.

Couper, Fiona J., and Barry K. Logan. "Drugs and Human Performance Fact Sheets." Washington, D.C.: National Highway Safety and Traffic Administration Report, August 2000.

Cravey, R H., and R.C. Baselt. "Forensic Toxicology." In Casarett, L.J., and J. Doull (eds.). *Toxicology: The Basic Science of Poisons.* New York: Macmillan, 1975, pp. 667–682.

"Creatine and Androstenedione—Two 'Dietary Supplements'." *The Medical Letter on Drugs and Therapeutics* 40:1039 (1998): 105–106.

Dafters, R.I., and E. Lynch. "Persistent Loss of Thermoregulation in the Rate Induced by 3,4-Methylenedioxymethamphetamine (MDMA or 'Ecstasy') but Not by Fenfluramine." *Psychopharmacology* 138 (1998): 207–212.

Drummer, O.H. *Forensic Aspects of Drugs of Abuse.* New York: Oxford University Press, 2001.

Edwards, R.W., and E.R. Oetting. "Inhalant Use in the United States." In Kozel, N., Z. Sloboda, and M. De La Rosa, eds. *Epidemiology of Inhalant Abuse: An International Perspective. National Institute on Drug Abuse Research Monograph 148.* DHHS Publication No. NIH 95-3831. Bethesda, Md.: National Institute on Drug Abuse, 1995.

Elliot, D., and L. Goldberg. "Intervention and Prevention of Steroid Use in Adolescents." *American Journal of Sports Medicine* 24:6 (1996): S46–S47.

Fendrich, M., M.E. Mackesy-Amiti, J.S. Wislar, and P.J. Goldstein. "Childhood Abuse and the Use of Inhalants: Differences by Degree of Use." *American Journal of Public Health* 87:5 (1997): 765–769.

Foltin, R.W., M.W. Fischman, J.J. Pedroso, and G.D. Pearlson. "Marijuana and Cocaine Interactions in Humans: Cardiovascular Consequences." *Pharmacology Biochemistry and Behavior* 28:4 (1987): 459–464.

French, E.D. "Delta-9 THC Excites ret VTA Dopamine Neurons Through Activation of Cannabinoid CB1 but Not Opioid Receptors." *Neuroscience Letters* 226 (1997): 159–162.

Garriott J. *Medicolegal Aspects of Alcohol Determination in Biological Specimens.* Littleton, Mass.: PSG Publishing, 1988.

Bibliography

Glaister, J. *The Power of Poison*. New York: William Morrow, 1954, pp. 153–182.

Gold, Mark S. "Cocaine (and Crack): Clinical Aspects." In Lowinson, ed. *Substance Abuse: A Comprehensive Textbook*, 3rd edition. Baltimore, Md.: Williams & Wilkins, 1997.

Goldberg, L., et al. "Anabolic Steroid Education and Adolescents: Do Scare Tactics Work?" *Pediatrics* 87:3 (1991): 283–286.

Goldberg, L., et al. "Effects of a Multidimensional Anabolic Steroid Prevention Intervention: The Adolescents Training and Learning to Avoid Steroids (ATLAS) Program." *Journal of the American Medical Association* 276:19 (1996): 1555–1562.

Goldberg, L., et al. "The ATLAS Program: Preventing Drug Use and Promoting Health Behaviors." *Archives of Pediatrics and Adolescent Medicine* 154 (2000): 332–338.

Goldstein, A. "Heroin Addiction: Neurology, Pharmacology, and Policy." *Journal of Psychoactive Drugs* 23:2 (1991): 123–133.

Gruber, A.J., and H.G. Pope, Jr. "Compulsive Weight Lifting and Anabolic Drug Abuse Among Women Rape Victims." *Comprehensive Psychiatry* 40:4 (1999): 273–277.

Gruber, A.J., and H.G. Pope, Jr. "Psychiatric and Medical Effects of Anabolic-androgenic Steroid Use in Women." *Psychotherapy and Psychosomatics* 69 (2000): 19–26.

Heishman, S.J., K. Arasteh, and M.L. Stitzer. "Comparative Effects of Alcohol and Marijuana on Mood, Memory, and Performance." *Pharmacology Biochemistry and Behavior* 58:1 (1997): 93–101.

Hoberman, J.M., and C.E. Yesalis. "The History of Synthetic Testosterone." *Scientific American* 272:2 (1995): 76–81.

Hofmann, A. *LSD: My Problem Child*. New York: McGraw-Hill, 1980.

Houts, M., R.C. Baselt, and R.H. Cravey. *Courtroom Toxicology*. New York: Matthew Bender, 1981.

Hughes, P.H., and O. Rieche. "Heroin Epidemics Revisited." *Epidemiology Review* 17:1 (1995): 66–73.

Jansson, L.M., D. Svikis, J. Lee, et al. "Pregnancy and Addiction: A Comprehensive Care Model." *Journal of Substance Abuse Treatment* 13:4 (1996): 321–329.

Javitt, D.C., and S.R. Zukin. "Recent Advances in the Phencyclidine Model of Schizophrenia." *American Journal of Psychiatry* 148 (1991): 1301–1308.

Karch, S. *Drug Abuse Handbook.* New York: CRC Press, 1998.

Kish, S.J., Y. Furukawa, L. Ang, et al. "Striatal Serotonin Is Depleted in Brain of a Human MDMA (Ecstasy) User." *Neurology* 55 (2000): 294–296.

Knight, B. "Ricin—A Potent Homicidal Poison." *British Medical Journal* 1 (1979): 350.

Koprich, J.B., E.-Y. Chen, N.M. Kanaan, et al. "Prenatal 3,4-Methylenedioxymethamphetamine (Ecstasy) Alters Exploratory Behavior, Reduces Monoamine Metabolism, and Increases Forebrain Tyrosine Hydroxylase Fiber Density of Juvenile Rats." *Neurotoxicology and Teratology* 25 (2003): 509–517.

Kornetsky, C. "Action of Opioid on the Brain-reward System." In Rapaka, R.S., and H. Sorer, eds. *Discovery of Novel Opioid Medications.* National Institute on Drug Abuse Research Monograph 147. NIH Publication No. 95-3887. Bethesda, MD: National Institute on Drug Abuse, 1991.

Lane, B. *The Encyclopaedia of Forensic Science.* London: Magpie Books, 2004.

Leder, B.Z., et al. "Oral Androstenedione Administration and Serum Testosterone Concentrations in Young Men." *Journal of the American Medical Association* 283:6 (2000): 779–782.

Lester, S.J., M. Baggott, S. Welm, et al. "Cardiovascular Effects of 3,4-Methylenedioxymethamphetamine: A Double-blind, Placebo-controlled Trial." *Annals of Internal Medicine* 133 (2000): 969–973.

Levine, B. *Principles of Forensic Toxicology.* Washington, D.C.: AAAC Press, 2003.

Liechti, M.E., and F.X. Vollenweider. "Which Neuroreceptors Mediate the Subjective Effects of MDMA in Humans? A Summary of Mechanistic Studies." *Human Psychopharmacology* 16 (2001): 589–598.

Lyles, J., and J.L. Cadet. "Methylenedioxymethamphetamine (MDMA, Ecstasy) Neurotoxicity: Cellular and Molecular Mechanisms." *Brain Research Reviews* 42 (2003): 155–168.

Bibliography

"Mandatory Guidelines for Federal Workplace Drug Testing Programs."
Federal Register notice (69 FR 19644) published April 13, 2004; effective
November 1, 2004.

Mason, A.P., and A.J. McBay. "Ethanol, Marijuana, and Other Drug Use in 600
Drivers Killed in Single-vehicle Crashes in North Carolina, 1978–1981."
Journal of Forensic Science 29:4 (1984): 987–1026.

Mathias, R. "Like Methamphetamine, Ecstasy May Cause Long-Term Brain
Damage." *NIDA Notes* 11 (1996): 7.

McCann, U.D., V. Eligulashvili, and G.A. Ricaurte. "(±)3,4-Methylenedioxy-
methamphetamine ('Ecstasy')–induced Serotonin Neurotoxicity: Clinical
Studies." *Neuropsychobiology* 42 (2000): 11–16.

Middleman, A.B., et al. "High-risk Behaviors Among High School Students
in Massachusetts Who Use Anabolic Steroids." *Pediatrics* 96:2 (1995):
268–272.

Mokdad, A.H., J.S. Marks, D.F. Stroup;, and J.L. Gerberding. "Actual Causes
of Death in the United States, 2000." *Journal of the American Medical
Association* 291 (2004): 1238–1245.

Morgan, M.J. "Ecstasy (MDMA): A Review of Its Possible Persistent
Psychological Effects." *Psychopharmacology* 152 (2000): 230–248.

Morgan, M.J. "Memory Deficits Associated with Recreational Use of 'Ecstasy'
(MDMA)." *Psychopharmacology* 141 (1999): 30–36.

"Multistage Outbreak of Poisonings Associated with Illicit Use of Gamma
Hydroxy Butyrate." *Morbidity and Mortality Weekly Report* 39:47 (1990):
861–863.

National Highway Traffic Safety Administration (NHTSA). "Marijuana and
Alcohol Combined Severely Impede Driving Performance." *Annals of
Emergency Medicine* 35:4 (2000): 398–399.

National Institute on Drug Abuse. *Epidemiologic Trends in Drug Abuse:
Advance Report, Community Epidemiology Work Group.* NIH Publication
No. 03-5363A. Bethesda, Md.: National Institute on Drug Abuse, 2003.

National Institute on Drug Abuse. *Epidemiologic Trends in Drug Abuse: Vol.
I. Highlights and Executive Summary of the Community Epidemiology*

Work Group, June 2001. NIH Publication No. 01-4916A. Bethesda, Md.: National Institute on Drug Abuse, 2001.

National Institute on Drug Abuse. *Epidemiologic Trends in Drug Abuse: Vol. II. Proceedings of the Community Epidemiology Work Group, June 2001.* NIH Publication No. 01-4917A. Bethesda, Md.: National Institute on Drug Abuse, 2001.

National Institute on Drug Abuse. *Epidemiologic Trends in Drug Abuse, Vol. II, Proceedings of the Community Epidemiology Work Group, December 2003.* NIH Publication No. 04-5365. Bethesda, Md.: National Institute on Drug Abuse, 2004.

National Institute on Drug Abuse. *Monitoring the Future, National Results on Adolescent Drug Use, Overview of Key Findings 2004.* NIH Publication No. 05-5726. Bethesda, Md.: National Institute on Drug Abuse, 2005.

National Institute on Drug Abuse. *Monitoring the Future: National Results on Adolescent Drug Use 2004.* Bethesda, Md.: National Institute on Drug Abuse, 2004.

National Institute on Drug Abuse. *National Survey Results on Drug Use From the Monitoring the Future Study, 1975–1994, Vol. I: Secondary School Students.* NIH Publication No. 93-3498. Bethesda, Md.: National Institute on Drug Abuse, 1995.

National Institute on Drug Abuse. *National Survey Results on Drug Use From the Monitoring the Future Study, 1975–1994, Vol. II: College Students and Young Adults.* NIH Publication No. 96-4027. Bethesda, Md.: National Institute on Drug Abuse, 1995.

National Institute on Drug Abuse. *National Survey Results on Drug Use From the Monitoring the Future Survey, 2003.* Bethesda, Md.: National Institute on Drug Abuse, 2003.

National Institute on Drug Abuse. *National Survey Results on Drug Use From the Monitoring the Future Study, 2004.* Bethesda, Md.: National Institute on Drug Abuse, 2004.

National Institute on Drug Abuse. *NIDA Capsule, Heroin.* Bethesda, Md.: National Institute on Drug Abuse, 1986.

Bibliography

National Institute on Drug Abuse. *NIDA Capsule, Methamphetamine Abuse.* Bethesda, Md.: National Institute on Drug Abuse, 1997.

National Institute on Drug Abuse. *NIDA InfoFacts, Crack and Cocaine, 1998.* Bethesda, Md.: National Institute on Drug Abuse, 1998.

National Institute on Drug Abuse. *NIDA InfoFacts, Inhalants.* Bethesda, Md.: National Institute on Drug Abuse, 2004.

National Institute on Drug Abuse. *Research Monograph 106.* Bethesda, Md.: National Institute on Drug Abuse, 1991, pp. 245–266.

"National Methamphetamine Strategy." Washington, D.C.: U.S. Department of Justice, 1996.

Obrocki, J., R. Buchert, O. Väterlein, et al. "Ecstasy—Long-term Effects on the Human Central Nervous System Revealed by Positron Emission Tomography." *British Journal of Psychiatry* 175 (1999): 186–188.

Office of National Drug Control Policy. *Heroin Facts and Figures.* Rockville, Md.: Office of National Drug Control Policy, 2004.

Office of National Drug Control Policy. *The National Drug Control Strategy: A Ten-Year Plan.* Rockville, Md.: Office of National Drug Control Policy, 1998.

Ohlsson, A., J.E. Lindgren, A. Wahlen, et al. "Plasma Delta-9 Tetrahydrocannabinol Concentrations and Clinical Effects After Oral and Intravenous Administration and Smoking." *Clinical and Pharmacological Therapy* 28:3 (1980): 409–416.

Parrott, A.C., and J. Lasky. "Ecstasy (MDMA) Effect upon Mood and Cognition: Before, During and After a Saturday Night Dance." *Psychopharmacology* 139 (1998): 261–268.

Pope, H.G., Jr., E.M. Kouri, and M.D. Hudson. "Effects of Supraphysiologic Doses of Testosterone on Mood and Aggression in Normal Men." *Archives of General Psychiatry* 57:2 (2000): 133–140.

Porcerelli, J.H., and B.A. Sandler. "Anabolic-androgenic Steroid Abuse and Psychopathology." *Psychiatric Clinics of North America* 21:4 (1998): 829–833.

Reneman, L., J. Booij, B. Schmand, et al. "Memory Disturbances in 'Ecstasy' Users are Correlated with an Altered Brain Serotonin Neurotransmission." *Psychopharmacology* 148 (2000): 322–324.

Rosenberg, N.L., et al. "Neuropsychologic Impairment and MRI Abnormalities Associated with Chronic Solvent Abuse." *Journal of Toxicology—Clinical Toxicology* 40:1 (2002): 21–34.

Schenk, S., D. Gittings, M. Johnstone, and E. Daniela. "Development, Maintenance and Temporal Pattern of Self-administration Maintained by Ecstasy (MDMA) in Rats." *Psychopharmacology* 169 (2003): 21–27.

Sharp, C.W., and N.L. Rosenberg. "Inhalants." In Lowinson, J.H., P. Ruiz, R.B. Millman, and J.G. Langrod, eds. *Substance Abuse: A Comprehensive Textbook*, 3rd edition. Baltimore: Williams and Wilkins, 1996, pp. 246–264.

Sharp, C.W., and N. L. Rosenberg. "Inhalant-related Disorders." In Tasman, A., J. Kay, and J.A. Lieberman, eds. *Psychiatry, Vol. 1*. Philadelphia: W.B. Saunders, 1997, pp. 835–852.

Sherlock, K., K. Wolff, A.W. Hay, and M. Conner. "Analysis of Illicit Ecstasy Tablets." *Journal of Accident and Emergency Medicine* 16 (1999): 194–197.

Shoptaw, S., et al. "Randomized Placebo-controlled Trial of Baclofen for Cocaine Dependence: Preliminary Effects for Individuals with Chronic Patterns of Cocaine Use." *Journal of Clinical Psychiatry* 64:12 (2003): 1440–1448.

Smith, S. "Poisons and Poisoners Through the Ages." *Medico-Legal Journal* 20 (1952): 153–166.

Snyder, Solomon H. *Drugs and the Brain.* New York: Scientific American Library, 1996, pp. 122–130.

Stewart, C.P., and A. Stolman, eds. *Toxicology, Mechanisms and Analytical Methods, Vol. 1.* New York: Academic Press, 1961, pp. 1–18.

Su, T.-P., et al. "Neuropsychiatric Effects of Anabolic Steroids in Male Normal Volunteers." *Journal of the American Medical Association* 269:21 (1993): 2760–2764.

Substance Abuse and Mental Health Services Administration (SAMHSA). *National Survey on Drug Use and Health.* Rockville, Md.: SAMHSA, 2002.

Substance Abuse and Mental Health Services Administration (SAMHSA). *National Findings From the 2003 National Survey on Drug Use and Health.* Rockville, Md.: SAMHSA, 2003.

Bibliography

Substance Abuse and Mental Health Services Administration (SAMHSA), Office of Applied Studies. *Drug Abuse Warning Network, 2003: Interim National Estimates of Drug-Related Emergency Department Visits.* DAWN Series D-26, DHHS Publication No. (SMA)04-3972. Rockville, Md.: SAMHSA, 2004.

Substance Abuse and Mental Health Services Administration (SAMHSA), Office of Applied Studies. *Emergency Department Trends from the Drug Abuse Warning Network, Final Estimates 1995–2002.* DHHS Publication No. (SMA)63-3780. Rockville, Md.: SAMHSA, 2003.

Substance Abuse and Mental Health Services Administration (SAMHSA). *Results from the 2003 National Survey on Drug Use and Health: National Findings.* NSDUH Series H-25. DHHS Publication No. (SMA)04-3964. Rockville, Md.: Department of Health and Human Services, 2004.

Substance Abuse and Mental Health Services Administration (SAMHSA), Office of Applied Studies. *Drug Abuse Warning Network, 2003: Area Profiles of Drug-Related Mortality.* DAWN Series D-27, DHHS Publication No. (SMA)05-4023. Rockville, Md.: Department of Health and Human Services, 2005.

Sullivan, M.L., C.M. Martinez, P. Gennis, and E.J. Gallagher. "The Cardiac Toxicity of Anabolic Steroids." *Progress in Cardiovascular Diseases* 41:1 (1998): 1–15.

Thompson, M.R., K.M. Li, K.J. Clemens, et al. "Chronic Fluoxetine Treatment Partly Attenuates the Long-term Anxiety and Depressive Symptoms Induced by MDMA ('Ecstasy') in Rats." *Neuropsychopharmacology* 29:40 (2004): 694–704.

Trestrail, John Harris. *Criminal Poisoning: Investigational Guide for Law Enforcement, Toxicologist, Forensic Scientists and Attorneys.* Totowa, NJ: Humana Press, 2000.

Ungerleider, J.T., and R.N. Pechnick. "Hallucinogens." In Lowenstein, J.H., P. Ruiz, and R.B. Millman, eds. *Substance Abuse: A Comprehensive Textbook,* 2nd edition. Baltimore: Williams & Wilkins, 1992.

Verkes, R.J., H.J. Gijsman, M.S.M. Pieters, et al. "Cognitive Performance and Serotonergic Function in Users of Ecstasy." *Psychopharmacology* 153 (2001): 196–202.

Wareing, M., J.E. Fisk, and P.N. Murphy. "Working Memory Deficits in Current and Previous Users of MDMA ('Ecstasy')." *British Journal of Psychology* 91 (2000): 181–188.

Westveer, A.E., J.P. Jarvis, and C.J. Jensen III. "Homicidal Poisoning: The Silent Offense." *The FBI Law Enforcement Bulletin* (August 2004).

Williams, A.F., M.A. Peat, D.J. Crouch, et al. "Drugs in Fatally Injured Young Male Drivers." *Public Health Report* 100:1 (1985): 19–25.

Yesalis, C.E. "Trends in Anabolic-androgenic Steroid Use Among Adolescents." *Archives of Pediatrics and Adolescent Medicine* 151 (1997): 1197–1206.

Yesalis, C.E., N.J. Kennedy, A.N. Kopstein, and M.S. Bahrke. "Anabolic-androgenic Steroid Use in the United States." *Journal of the American Medical Association* 270:10 (1993): 1217–1221.

FURTHER READING

Emsley, J. *The Elements of Murder: A History of Poisons.* New York, Oxford University Press, 2005.

Evans, C. *The Casebook of Forensic Detection: How Science Solved 100 of the World's Most Baffling Crimes.* New York: John Wiley and Sons, 1996.

Farrell, M. *Poisons and Poisoners: An Encyclopedia of Homicidal Poisonings.* London: Robert Hale, 1992.

James, S.H., and J.J. Nordby. *Forensic Science: An Introduction to Scientific and Investigative Techniques.* Boca Raton, Fla.: CRC Press, 2002.

Kelleher, M.D., and C.L. Kelleher. *Murder Most Rare: The Female Serial Killer.* Westport, Conn.: Praeger, 1998.

Nash, J.R. *Encyclopedia of World Crime.* Wilmette, Ill.: Crime Books, 1990.

Pollack, O. *The Criminality of Women.* Westport Conn.: Greenwood Press, 1978.

Stevens, S.D., and A. Klarner. *Deadly Doses: A Writer's Guide to Poisons.* New York: Writer's Digest Books, 1990.

Web Sites

American Academy of Forensic Science
http://www.aafs.org

American Association of Poison Control Centers
http://www.aapcc.org

International Association of Forensic Toxicology
http://www.tiaft.org

National Capital Poison Center
http://www.poison.org

National Highway Traffic Safety Administration: Drugs and Human Performance Fact Sheets
http://www.nhtsa.dot.gov/PEOPLE/INJURY/research/job185drugs/index.htm

National Institute on Drug Abuse (NIDA)
http://www.nida.nih.gov

SAMHSA Alcohol and Drug Information

http://www.health.org/default.aspx

Schaffer Library of Drug Policy

http://www.druglibrary.org/schaffer/Misc/driving/contents.htm

Society of Forensic Toxicologists

http://soft-tox.org

World Anti-Doping Agency (WADA)

http://www.wada-ama.org/en/

PICTURE CREDITS

Index

ABOUT THE AUTHOR

Richard A. Stripp, Ph.D., is an assistant professor of forensic pharmacology and toxicology at The City University of New York John Jay College of Criminal Justice. In addition to his academic appointment, he has several years of experience as a practicing toxicologist at a medical examiners office and for the United States government. He currently serves as an expert toxicology consultant and has worked on several forensic cases related to drug and chemical effects on humans.

ABOUT THE EDITOR

Lawrence Kobilinsky, Ph.D., is a professor of biology and immunology at The City University of New York John Jay College of Criminal Justice. He currently serves as science advisor to the college's president and is also a member of the doctoral faculties of biochemistry and criminal justice of the CUNY Graduate Center. He is an advisor to forensic laboratories around the world and serves as a consultant to attorneys on major crime issues related to DNA analysis and crime scene investigation.